TECHNOLOGY BREAKTHROUGHS

12 BIGGEST BREAKTHROUGHS IN COVID-19 TECHNOLOGY

BLACK RABBIT BOOKS

JANIE SCHEFFER

Table of Contents

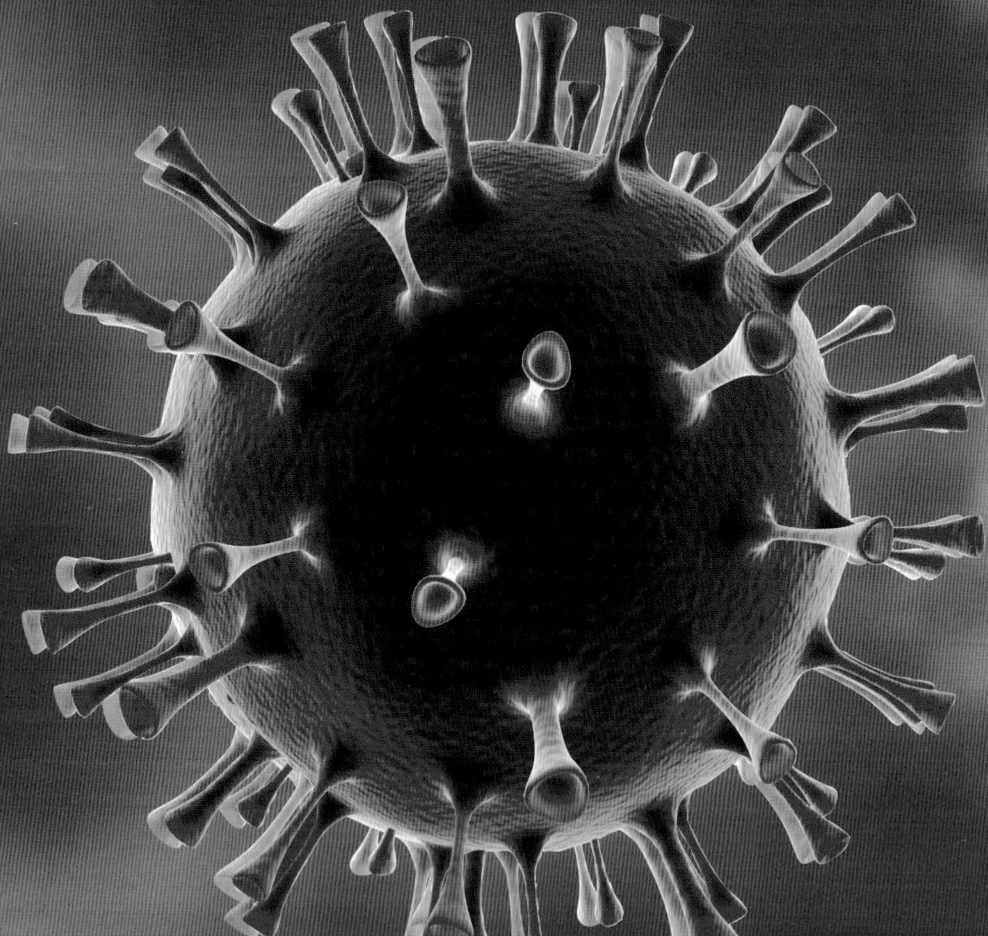

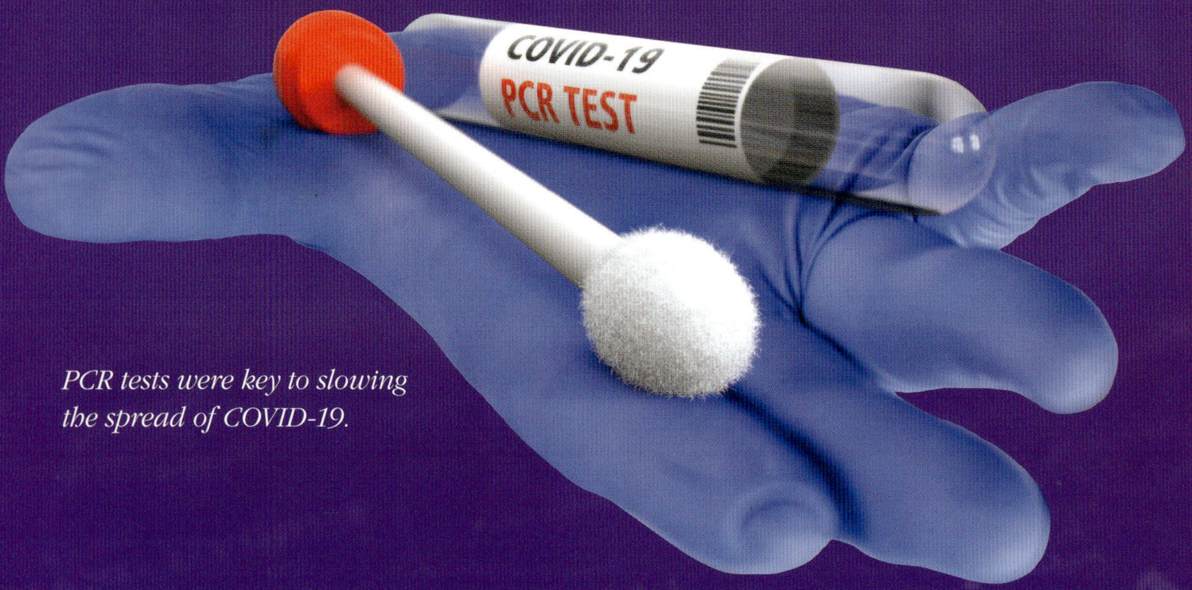

PCR tests were key to slowing the spread of COVID-19.

New Disease Drives *Viral Tests*

1

In 2019, a new disease started in China. It was named COVID-19. It caused people to have a fever and a cough. The sickness spread quickly.

Testing became important. A test would know to tell if a person was infected. The infected person could stay away from other people. This could help slow the spread. Scientists began their work. They learned about the virus behind the disease. It is called SARS-CoV-2. It is made of **genetic** material called RNA. Scientists needed a test to measure RNA.

Dr. Kary B. Mullis knew of a way to test RNA. He created the PCR method back in 1987. PCR copies genetic material. Once many copies are made, the matter is easier to study. It is also easier to measure.

PCR tests led the way to fast test lab cards pictured below.

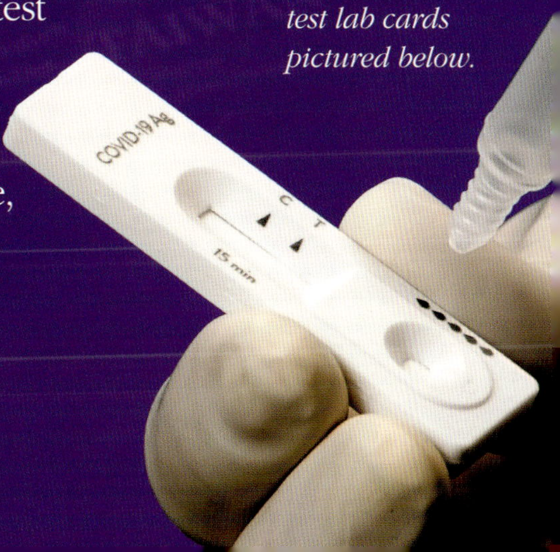

In early 2020, scientists used PCR. They followed Mullis' process. They added dye to help measure. Doctors looked for the virus' RNA in a person's body. They used a DNA sample from the patient's mouth or nose. DNA contains RNA. The PCR test copied the RNA. It used heat to make millions of copies. A positive result meant the virus' RNA was present in the sample. Early on, these tests were done in a lab. They were accurate but not quick. It could take days for a result.

Meanwhile, a California company was at work. Quidel Corporation makes health-care tests. It released a faster COVID-19 test in 2020. The power of this test was its speed. This new test gave results in minutes. The test checked a sample for proteins called **antigens**. They are found on the outside of the virus. If the test finds the proteins, then COVID-19 is present. The person knew they were infected and could keep away from others. The rapid tests were quick but not as accurate as PCR.

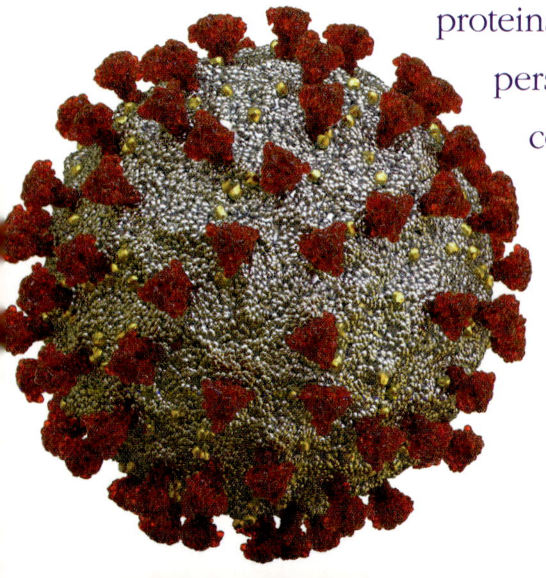

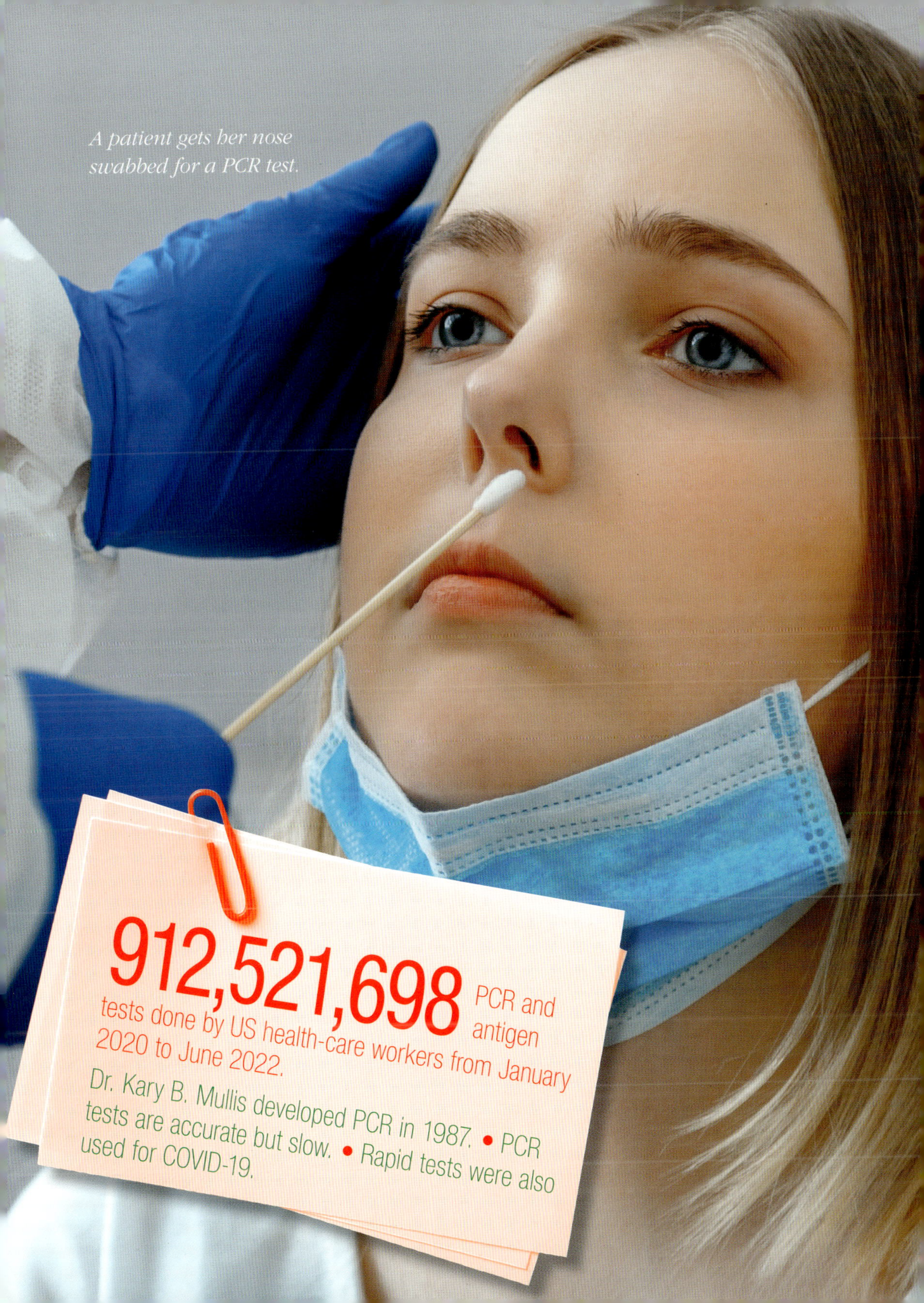

A patient gets her nose swabbed for a PCR test.

912,521,698 PCR and antigen tests done by US health-care workers from January 2020 to June 2022.

Dr. Kary B. Mullis developed PCR in 1987. • PCR tests are accurate but slow. • Rapid tests were also used for COVID-19.

Face Masks Help Limit *Disease Spread*

2

Protective masks have been around for a long time. They have helped slow the spread of illness. Louis Pasteur was a French chemist. In 1861, he made a discovery. He found bacteria in the air. Bacteria spread when someone talks, sneezes, or coughs. In the late 1890s, some surgeons started to wear face masks. The masks were simple. They were pieces of gauze tied with string. They covered the nose and mouth. These early masks protected patients. They kept a surgeon's germs from entering wounds.

In 1911, there was a **pandemic** in China. It was the Manchurian plague. About 60,000 people died. Dr. Wu Lien-teh was asked to help. He had studied medicine at Cambridge University. Wu found how the plague was spread. Most people thought it was fleas. But Wu figured out it spread through the air.

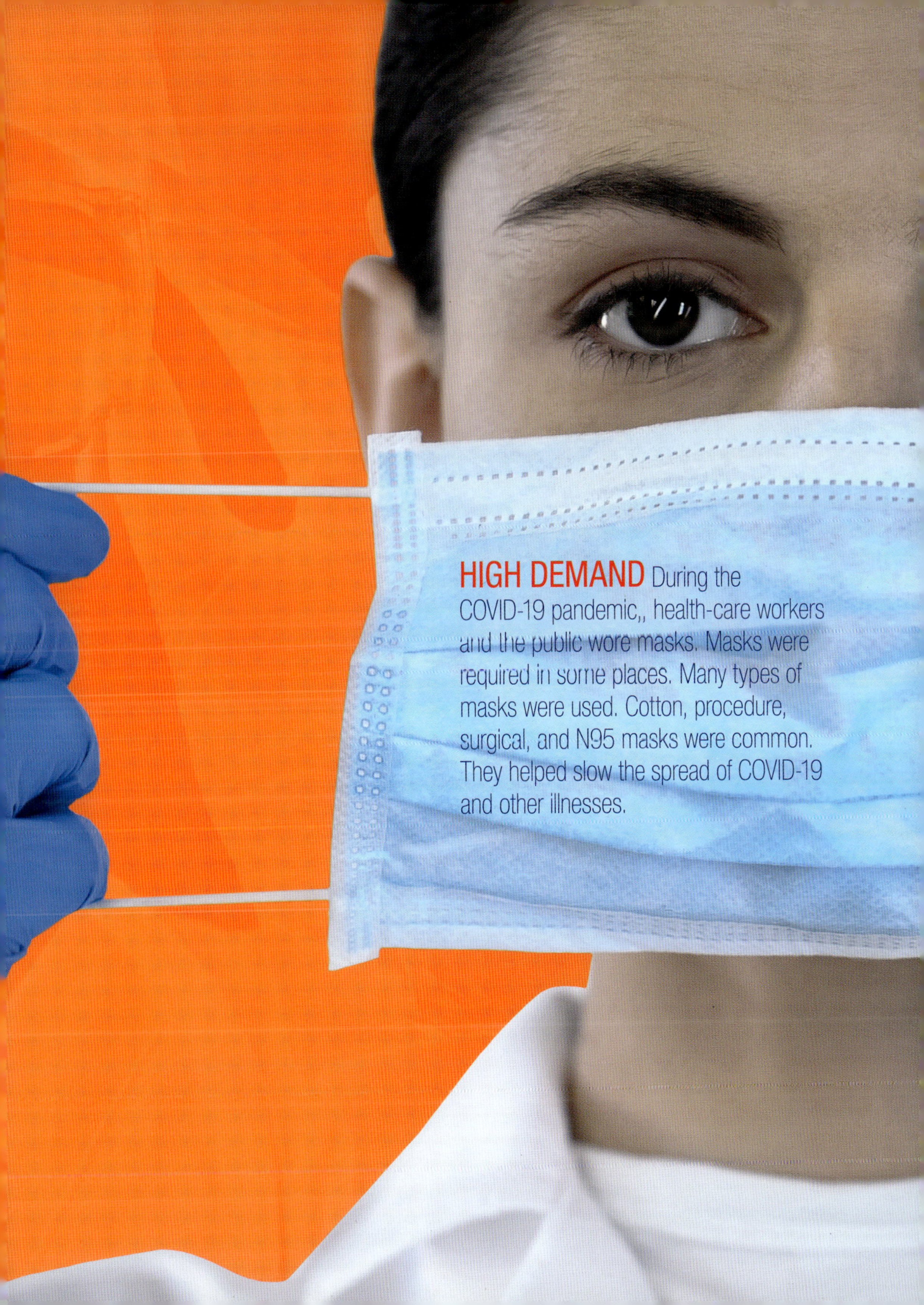

HIGH DEMAND During the COVID-19 pandemic,, health-care workers and the public wore masks. Masks were required in some places. Many types of masks were used. Cotton, procedure, surgical, and N95 masks were common. They helped slow the spread of COVID-19 and other illnesses.

60,000 The number of deaths caused by the Manchurian plague before Wu made his mask.

Dr. Wu Lien-teh's mask was simple. • The mask filtered the air. • His design led to disposable masks.

Wu made a new face mask. He layered pieces of gauze. Then he wrapped them in cotton. Wu added ties to each side. The ties went around a person's ears. Health-care workers wore Wu's masks. The public did too. The layers of gauze and cotton were an effective defense. They filtered the air. This protected a person from the plague bacteria. During the plague, masks were in high demand. Luckily, they were cheap to make. The materials were easy to get. Companies and the public could make them.

There have been many mask designs since 1911. Wu's mask led to a disposable mask in 1930. Disposable masks are made of paper. They are also made of synthetic material. By the 1960s, most masks were disposable. They were made to be worn only once. The throwaway masks kept hospitals clean. They also saved hospitals time and money.

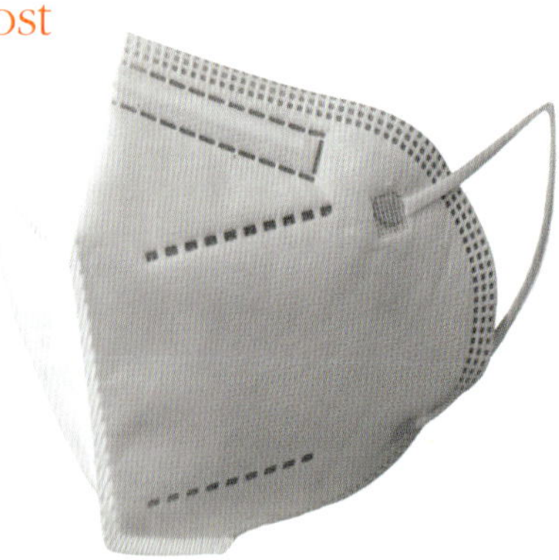

Respirators Filter Harmful *Particles*

3

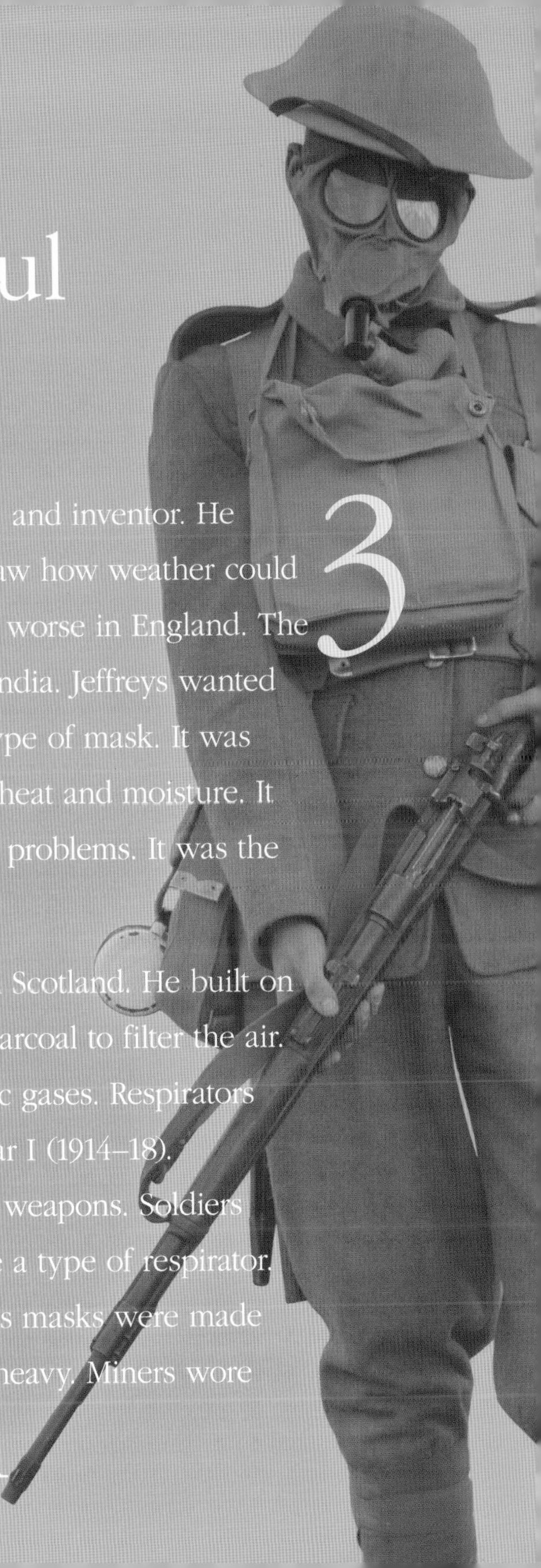

Julius Jeffreys was a surgeon, writer, and inventor. He moved from India to England. He saw how weather could affect health. His sister's asthma got worse in England. The country was colder and drier than India. Jeffreys wanted to help his sister. He made a new type of mask. It was finished in 1836. His mask trapped heat and moisture. It helped people with throat and lung problems. It was the world's first **respirator**.

John Stenhouse was a chemist from Scotland. He built on Jeffrey's design in 1854. He used charcoal to filter the air. This new respirator filtered out toxic gases. Respirators became important during World War I (1914–18). Dangerous chemicals were used as weapons. Soldiers wore gas masks. These masks were a type of respirator. They protected the soldiers. The gas masks were made of **fiberglass**. They were large and heavy. Miners wore

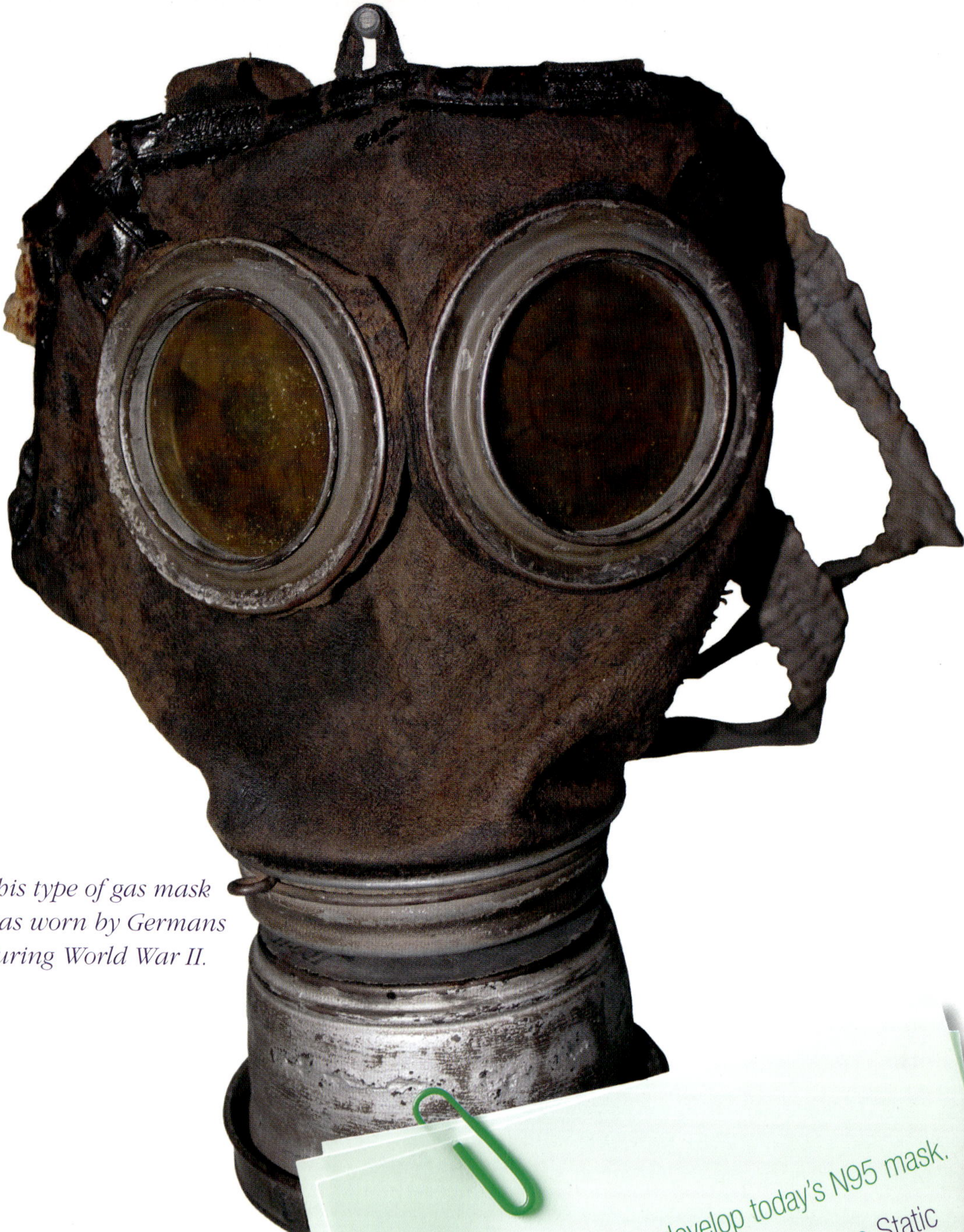

This type of gas mask was worn by Germans during World War II.

20 Years it took to develop today's N95 mask.

The first respirators were large and heavy. • Static charge pulled particles from the air. • N95s were first used by construction workers.

these gas masks too. They kept miners safe from black lung disease.

Smaller, lighter respirators were needed. Sara Little Turnbull was an American magazine editor. She was also a product designer. She made a mask from melted **polymers**. She took her discovery to 3M. The company uses science and technology to make products. Turnbull and 3M made a mask in 1961. It was meant for use in surgery. It had fiberglass filters. But it could not stop the spread of germs. So it became a dust mask. Turnbull and 3M took out the fiberglass filters. They tried material used in gift-wrapping ribbons. It worked. In 1972, the first N95 dust respirator was made.

Dr. Peter Tsai was a researcher and scientist. He was from Taiwan. He created an air filter made of plastic fibers. He added static electricity to the fibers. The static charge pulls particles out of the air. This includes dust and viruses. The particles cling to the filter. The air is cleaned. Tsai's new filter went into 3M's N95. These respirators went on the market in the 1990s. Construction workers were the first to use them. N95s filtered 95 percent of harmful particles.

Think About It The N95 filter was first made for home air filters. Its screens were for heating and cooling systems. Now the air filters protect health-care workers, especially during pandemics. Why do designs grow and change? What is another technology that has been given a new purpose?

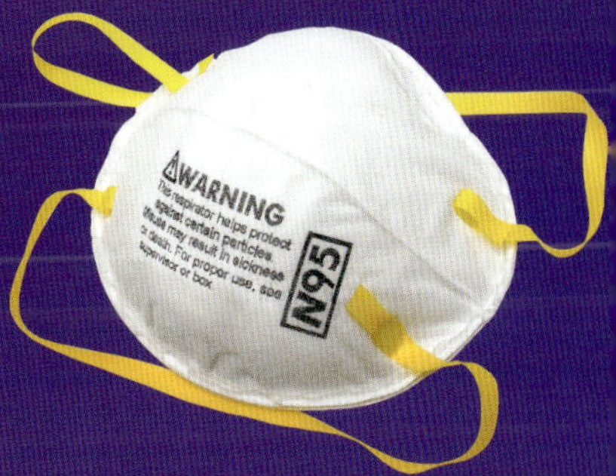

4

Sterilization Prevents *Infection*

COVID-19 spread around the world quickly. There was a rush of patients. Health-care workers tried to keep up. Equipment and tools had to be **sterilized**. Protective equipment like masks did too. An N95 was the best defense for nurses and doctors. But they could only be worn once. There was no approved technology to clean them. To make matters worse, there was a shortage of these masks. Finding a way to clean the masks became important. In 2020, the Food and Drug Administration (FDA) put out new guidances. It approved more cleaning systems for masks.

Advanced Sterilization Products (ASP) stepped up to help. ASP is a company in Maryland. It was started in 1987 by a group of Texas scientists. It builds systems that clean equipment and tools. The systems use hydrogen peroxide vapor and **plasma**. Together, the

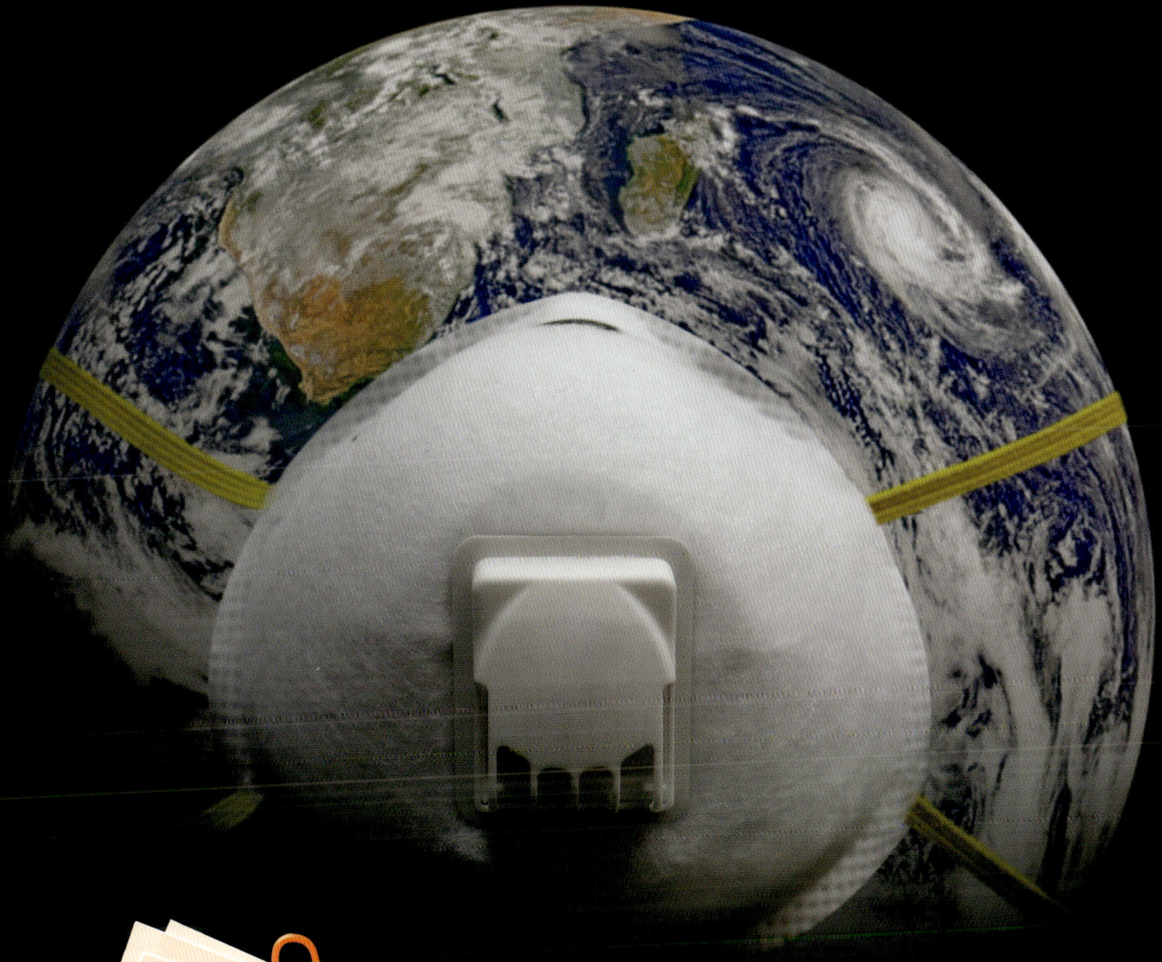

480 Number of N95 respirators cleaned daily by one ASP machine.

ASP worked with the FDA. • Each N95 could be cleaned twice. • ASP systems are used worldwide.

two substances are powerful. They clean medical equipment fully. They do not leave an unsafe coating.

The original system was approved by the FDA in 1993. Since then, two more systems have been created. In 2020, the FDA approved all three to be used during the pandemic. The ASP systems could clean an N95 two times. This extended the life of an N95. The respirators could be worn three times instead of only once. This helped save protective equipment during the shortage.

A nurse pulls out a tray of sterilized equipment.

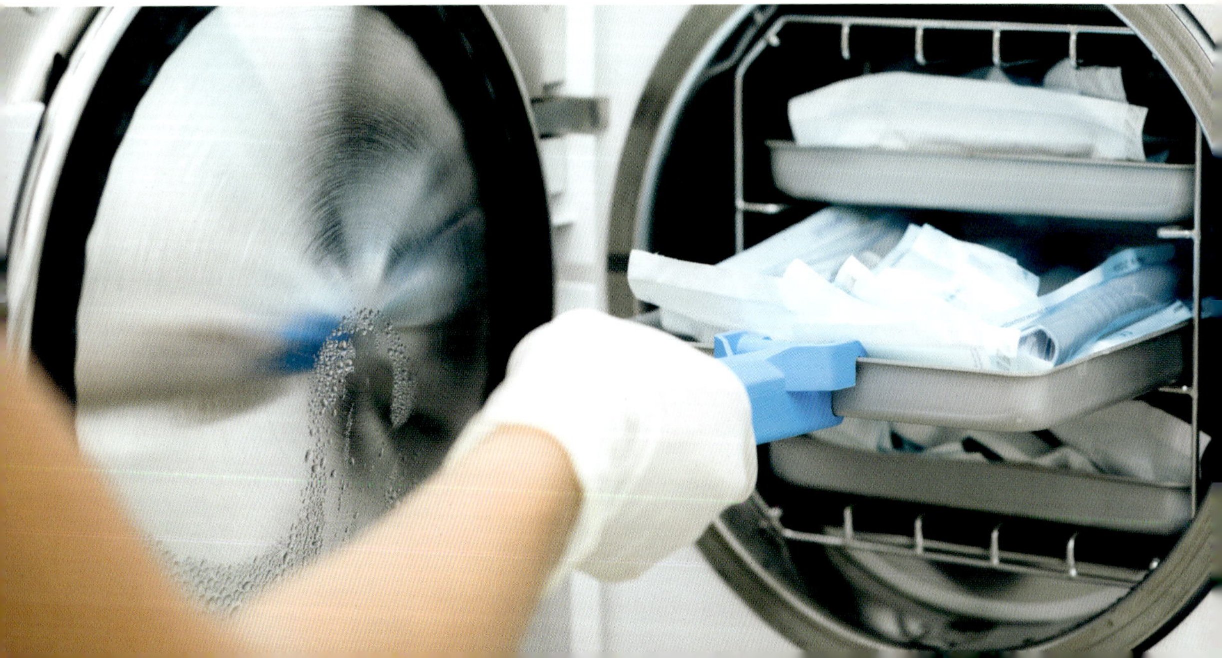

Ventilators Are a *Lifesaver*

5

Ventilators have existed for more than a century. They help people breathe. There are two types of machines. One type uses positive pressure. It pumps air directly into the lungs. This is positive pressure. The second type uses negative pressure. It works outside the body. The machine lowers the air pressure around the body to create a vacuum. The chest expands and pulls air into the lungs. Then the machine releases the air pressure. The chest deflates and the lungs exhale.

Inventor Johann Heinrich Drager was from Germany. In 1907, he and his son created the Pulmotor. It used the positive pressure with a face mask. It could force air into the lungs. It was the first model to do this.

Philip Drinker and Louis Agassiz Shaw made a new model in the 1920s. It was called the iron lung. It helped treat people with **polio**.

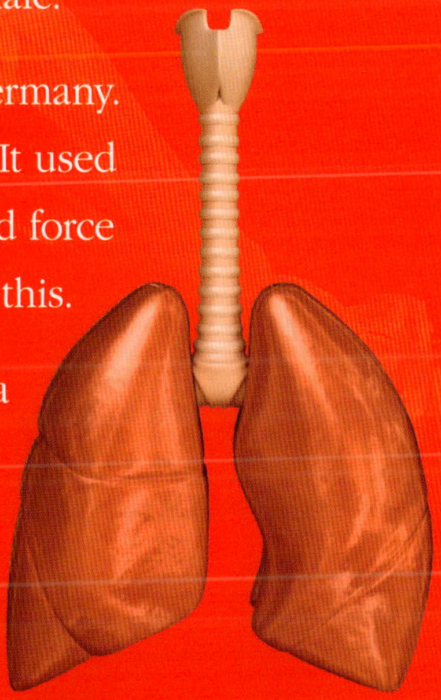

160,000 Total number of ventilators in the United States in 2020.

Ventilators have existed for more than a century. • Bird's model was the first to be mass-produced. • It helped COVID-19 patients breathe easier.

The iron lung worked by using negative pressure. The patient was enclosed in a large box from the neck down. It was airtight. **Bellows** pulled air out of the box. The air pressure lowered. It caused the patient's lungs to fill. Then bellows forced air back into the box. The air pressure grew. So air was forced out of the patient's lungs.

A model from 1958 led to today's ventilators. Dr. Forrest M. Bird was a US Army pilot and engineer. He worked on breathing devices for pilots. He invented the Bird Mark 7 Respirator. It helped patients with polio come out of the iron lung. The Bird Mark 7 was a positive pressure model. It forced air in and out of the lungs. The air traveled through a face mask. Bird's model was effective. It was not too expensive. It was also the first respirator to be **mass-produced**. Bird entered the Inventors Hall of Fame in 1995.

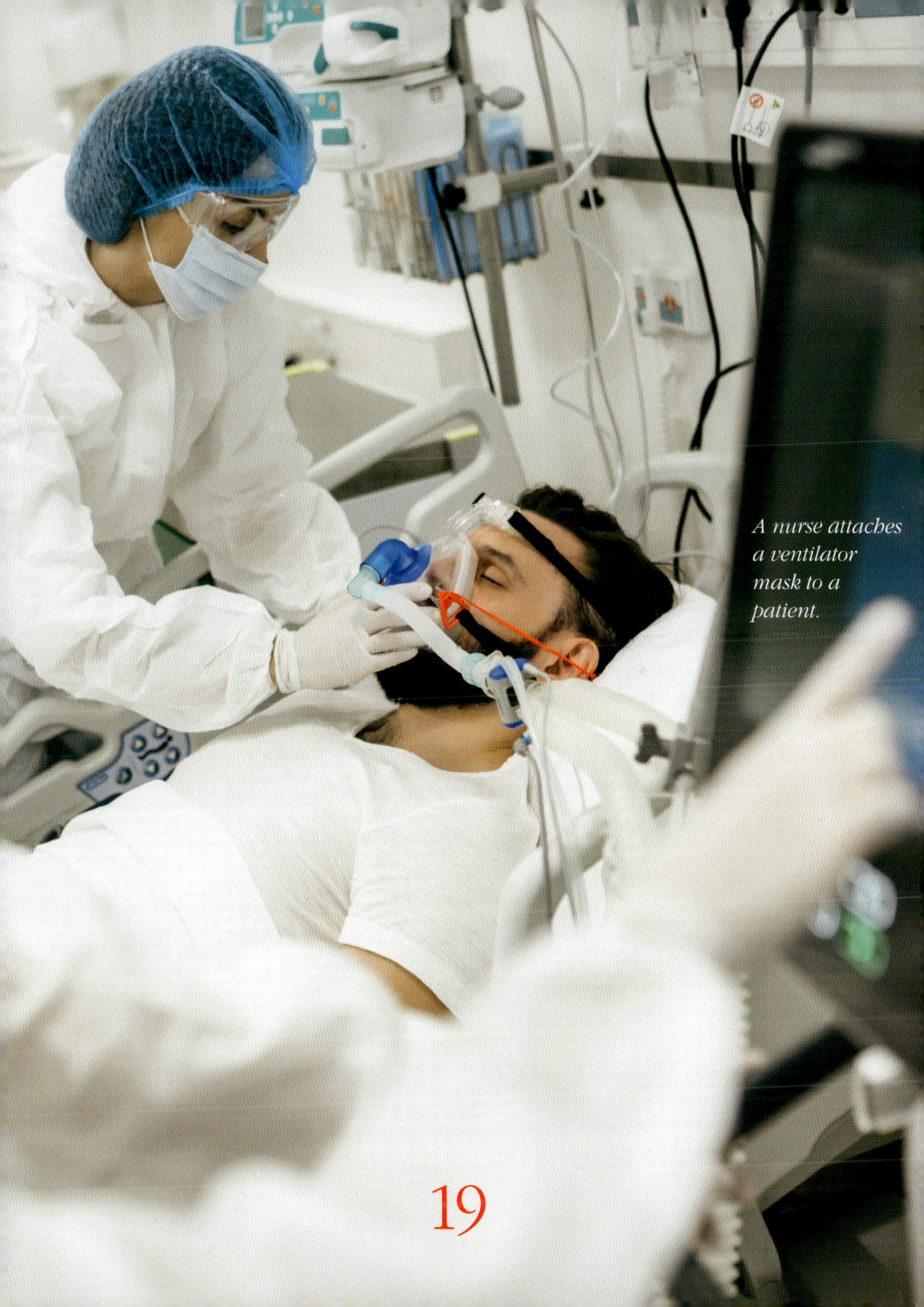

A nurse attaches a ventilator mask to a patient.

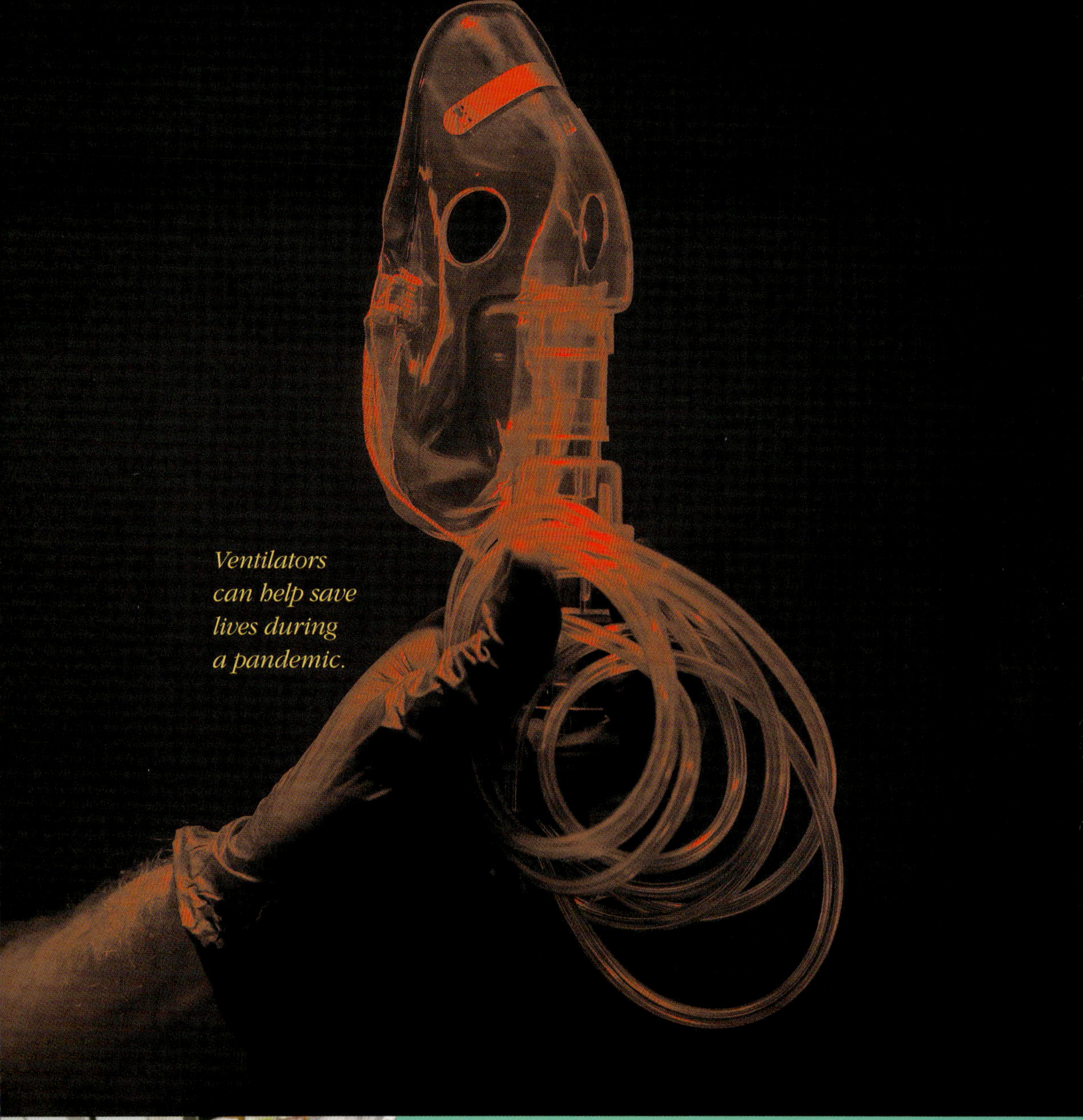

Ventilators can help save lives during a pandemic.

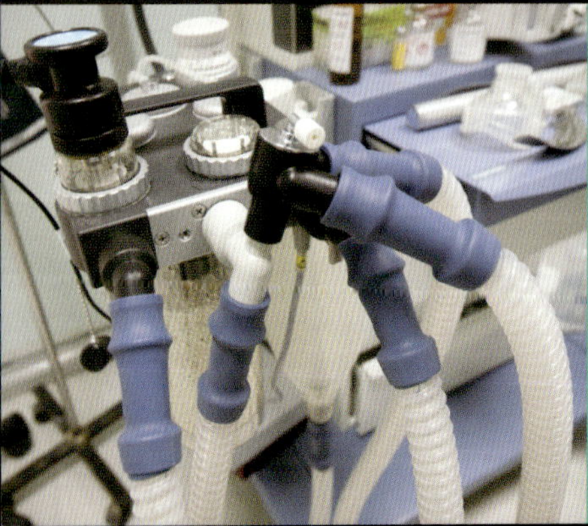

SPLITTERS COVID-19 caused breathing problems for many people. Ventilators were needed worldwide. In New York State alone, 30,000 were needed. Splitters helped with the problem. This technology already existed before COVID-19. Splitters divide the air flow. They also collect exhaled air. Splitters let two patients use one ventilator.

6

Telemedicine Provides *Care from Afar*

Telemedicine brings health care into the home. It began in the 1920s. Reverend John Flynn was from Australia. He started Aerial Medical Service (AMS). It used telegraphs and the radio. AMS doctors spoke with patients. Then they **diagnosed** and treated from afar. This was one of the first telemedicine services.

The 1950s brought about change. A television was used to monitor patients. Doctors could see a patient from a distance. In 1964, two health-care buildings were connected. They were 112 miles (180 kilometers) apart in Nebraska. They used a two-way video link. They were able to interact and communicate. In the 1990s, government funding improved telemedicine. The use of the internet did too.

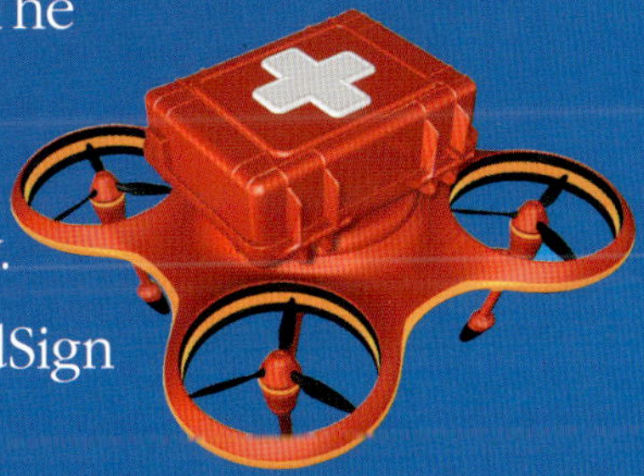

In a pandemic, exposure and spread are risky. Telemedicine can lower the risk. In 2020, MedSign made a new technology. The company's CEO, Tom Conroy, helped create Qortex. It is a health-care platform that uses the internet. It can be set up on a television. Doctors can both see and hear their patients. Qortex allows for round-the-clock virtual visits. And it tracks a patient's **vital signs**. Conroy designed it for his aging father.

Amwell also developed a new technology. In 2021, the US company released Converge. It is another health-care platform. It connects all parts of a patient's care. Virtual visits can happen on a smartphone or computer. Doctors are able to diagnose and treat. They can prescribe medication too. And the patient can be connected to their insurance. Care is offered 24 hours each day. The platform offers health education tools. It connects patients to health-care products. Patients can purchase exam kits to use at home.

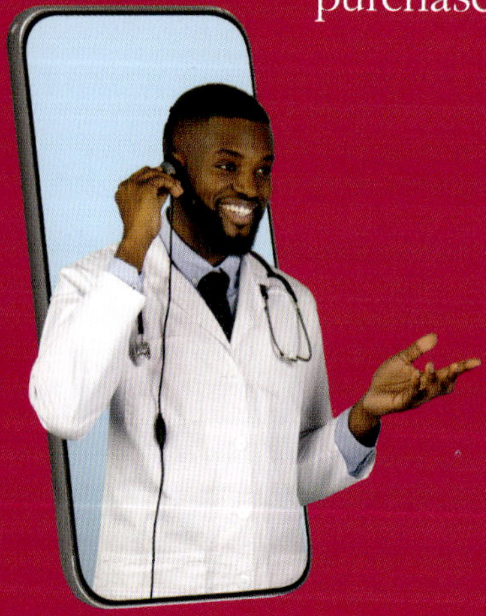

Think About It About half of health-care visits were virtual in 2020. Telemedicine is more common now than before COVID-19. What do you think are some pros and cons of telemedicine?

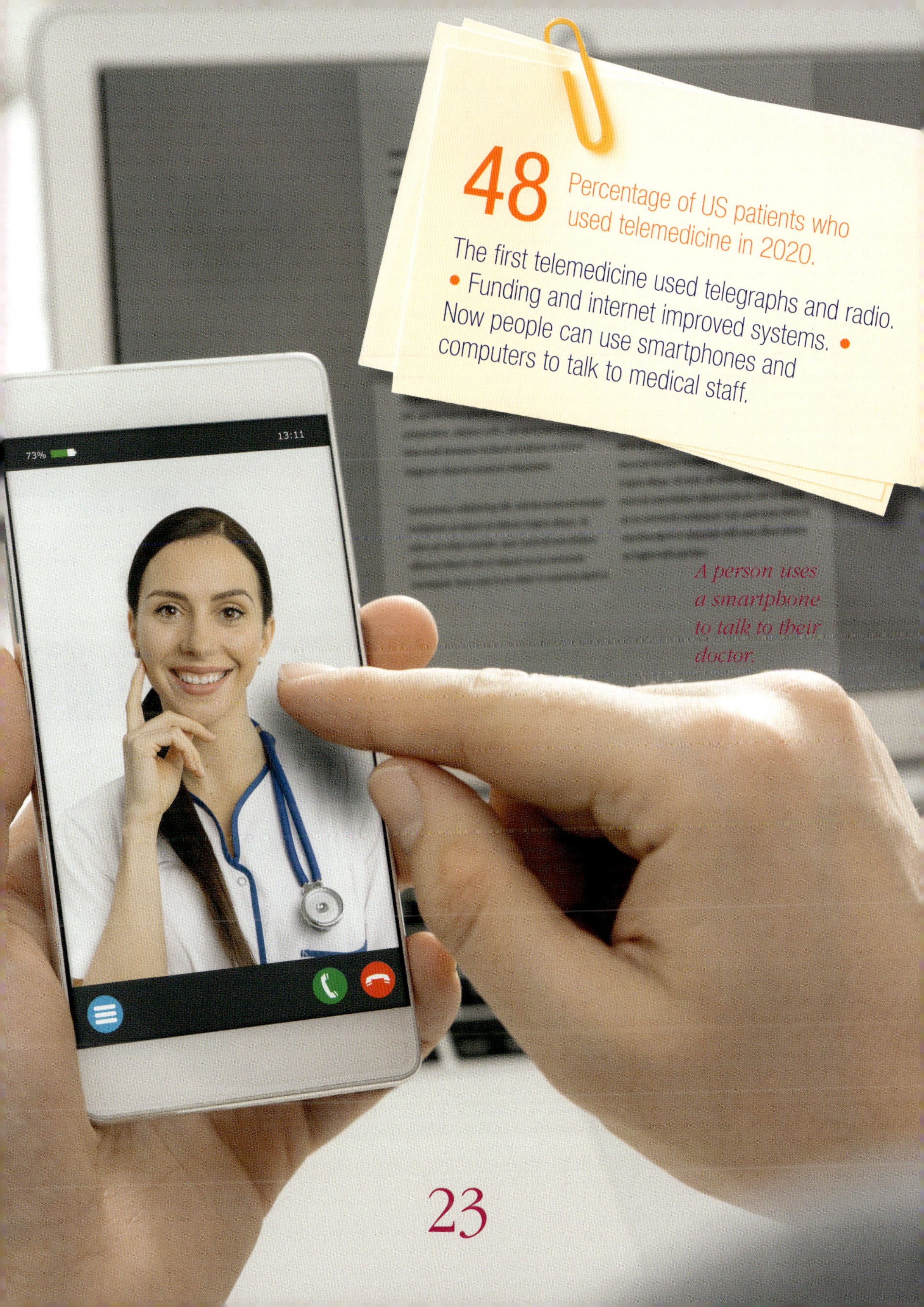

48 Percentage of US patients who used telemedicine in 2020.

The first telemedicine used telegraphs and radio. • Funding and internet improved systems. • Now people can use smartphones and computers to talk to medical staff.

A person uses a smartphone to talk to their doctor.

Antibody Test Indicates *Past Infection*

7 Another COVID-19 test was approved in 2020. It was made by a US biotech company called Cellex. They created an **antibody** test. An antibody is in the blood. It fights off viruses and bacteria. Each antibody fights a specific antigen. Cellex's test does not diagnose a person. Instead, it can tell if someone has already had COVID-19.

The test uses a blood sample. Blood is taken from the vein and sent to a lab. There, a few drops are put on a testing strip. The strip reacts to two antibodies. The body makes these specifically to fight off the COVID-19 virus. Results take about 15 to 20 minutes. A positive result means the person has had COVID-19 in the past few months. These results help scientists learn

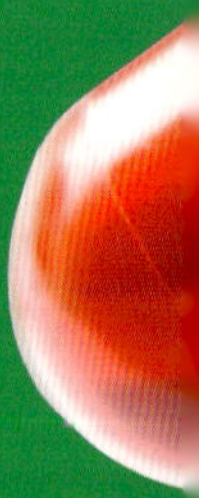

88 Number of different COVID-19 antibody tests approved by FDA as of September 2021.

Antibodies tell if the body has already fought a virus. • First tests needed a lab. • Faster tests came next.

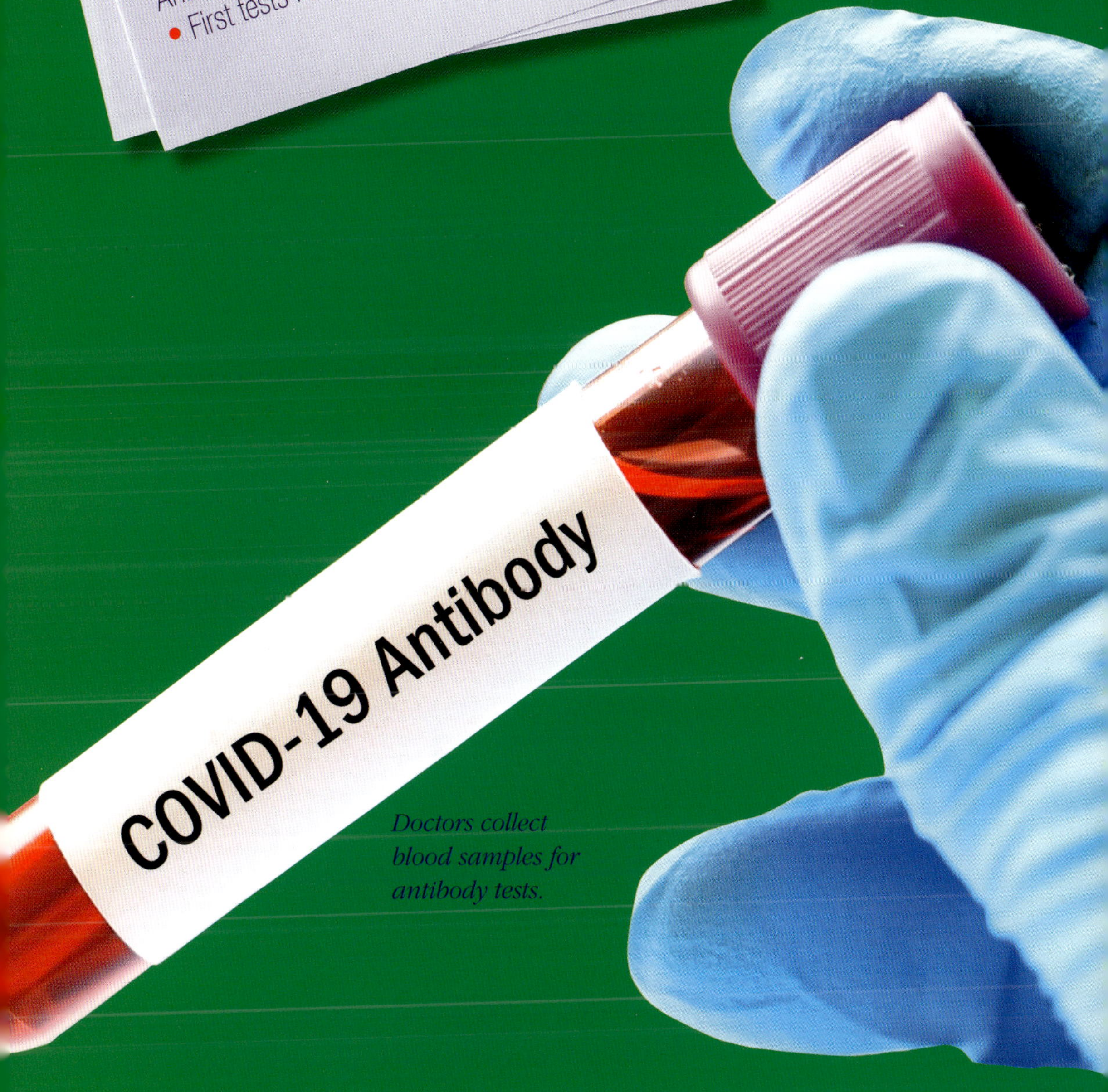

Doctors collect blood samples for antibody tests.

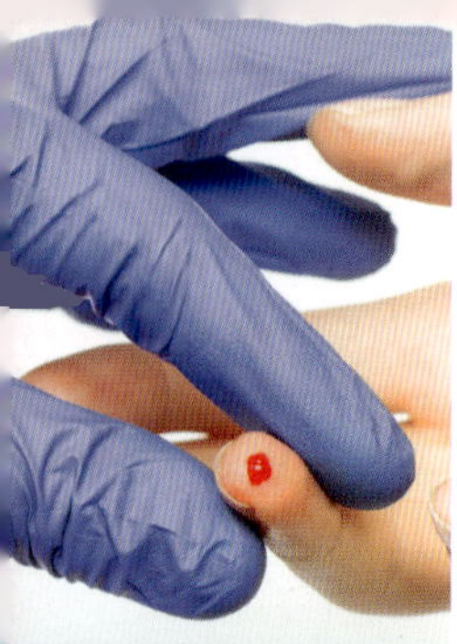

about the virus. They can show how the body reacted to the infection.

Cellex's test used lateral flow testing. This technology already existed, so it was easy to adapt to COVID-19. Another biotech company improved on Cellex's test. Assure Tech is based in China. Later in 2020, the FDA cleared its new antibody test. Like Cellex's test, it uses lateral flow. But Assure Tech uses just a finger prick for blood. It is a point-of-care test. This means it does not need to be sent to a lab. A person can receive the results right away.

IMPROVED TESTING Antibody testing does not prove **immunity**. Recent changes have improved antibody testing. Now tests can measure a patient's antibody levels. The levels can help explain someone's immune response.

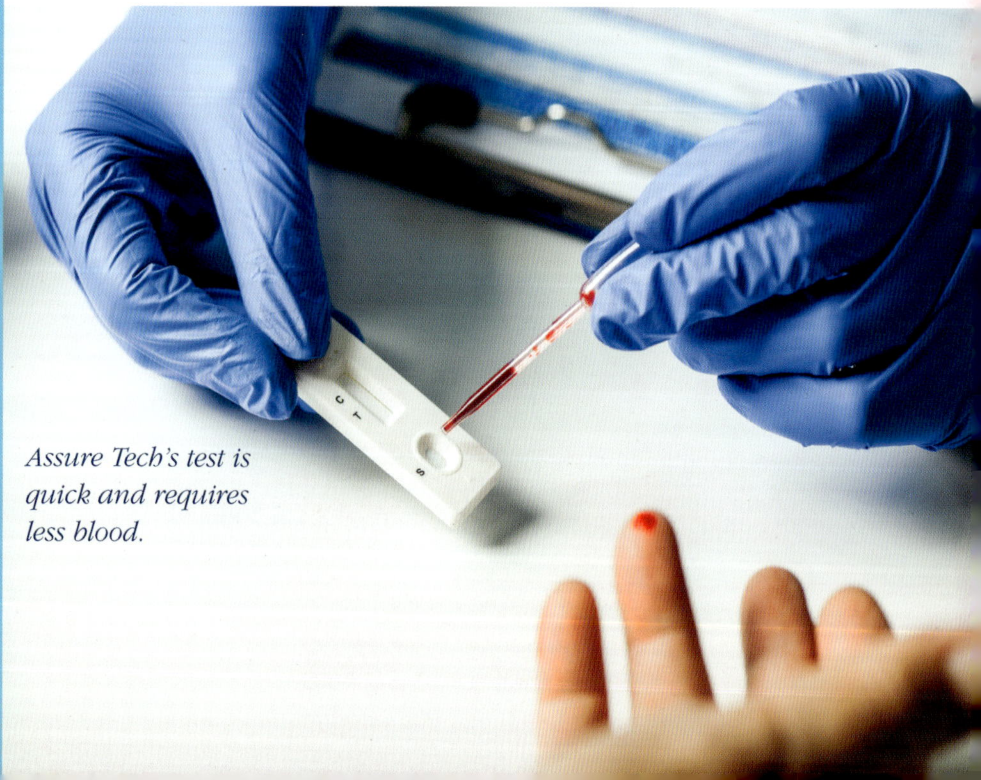

Assure Tech's test is quick and requires less blood.

At-Home Tests Give Results *Quickly*

8

Until November 2020, COVID-19 testing was only in health-care settings. Then, an at-home test was made. It changed the diagnosis process. A California company, Lucira, invented the first at-home COVID-19 test. Its test kit was approved by the FDA. People needed a prescription to get it. It is a molecular test. It looks for RNA. But it differs from PCR testing. It does not need high heat. It can copy genetic material at room temperature. The kit comes with a testing strip. A person swabs their nose. Then they place the swab in a vial of liquid and mix. They drop the liquid onto the testing strip. The strip detects the virus. Then the person waits for results. The whole test can be done in 30 minutes.

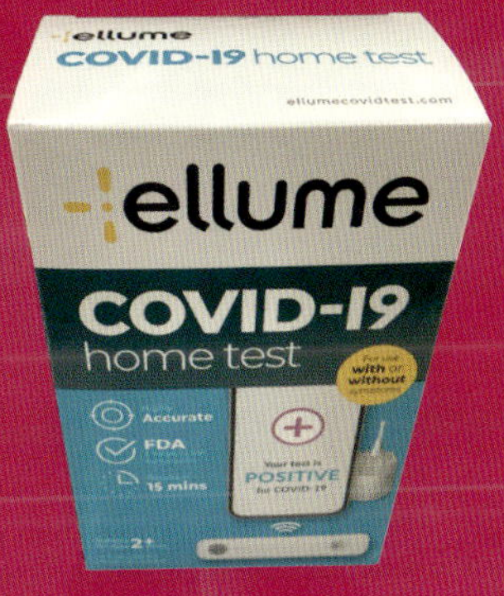

Ellume USA also created a home test. Dr. Sean Parsons founded Ellume. He started the company

10-20 Percent decrease in sensitivity of at-home tests. This is compared to PCR tests that are more accurate.

A prescription was needed for the first at-home tests. • The Ellume test used an app. • By 2022, tests were free and accessible.

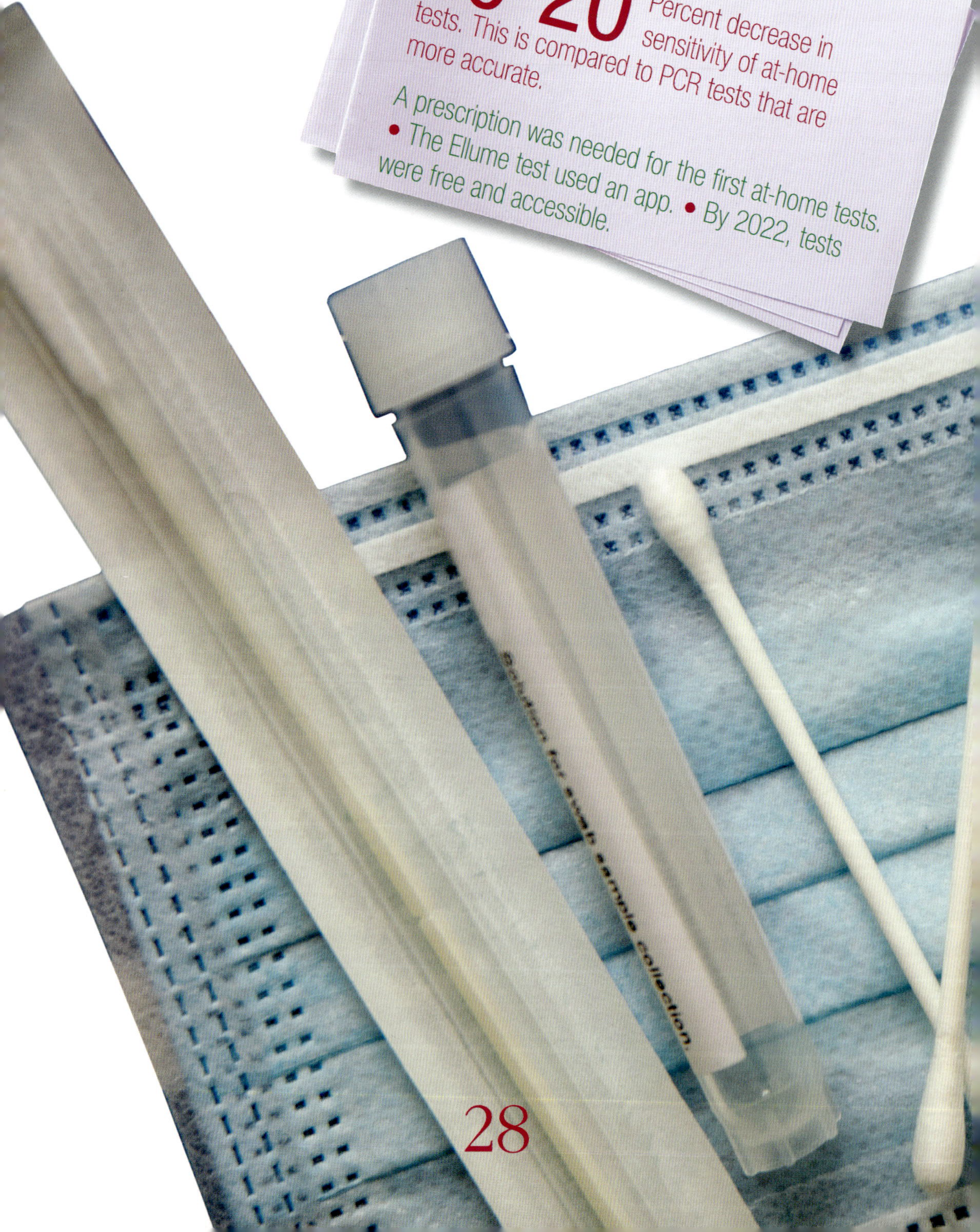

after the swine flu outbreak in 2009. The FDA cleared its COVID-19 test in December 2020. It is an antigen test. People do not need a prescription to get it. This made it more available to buy. The test also uses a nasal swab. The sample is placed onto the testing strip. The strip detects proteins. Results are given within 15 minutes on an app. The app also gives step-by-step intructions for testing.

By 2022, at-home COVID-19 tests were free. They were easy to come by. Results were ready quickly. A person with symptoms could act right away. They now knew when stay home. This helped slow the spread.

Think About It At-home COVID-19 tests have changed the diagnostic process. They have brought it into people's homes. How do you think at-home COVID-19 tests will impact future health testing?

Electronic Reporting Improves Control *and Response*

9

The Digital Bridge was started in 2016. It was created by a team of US government groups. Their goal was to easily share health information. Health-care systems and public health groups needed to communicate. They had to share information about widespread illness. And it needed to be shared quickly. It also needed to be correct. The Digital Bridge made this possible. The technology is electronic. It turns a disease report into an electronic case report (eCR). The eCR collects information about a patient. Age and diagnosis are collected. Test results are collected too. Then the Digital Bridge decides if the eCR is shared. If so, it is sent to public health groups.

eCR became a main focus for the pandemic. It provided important information about COVID-19's spread. It

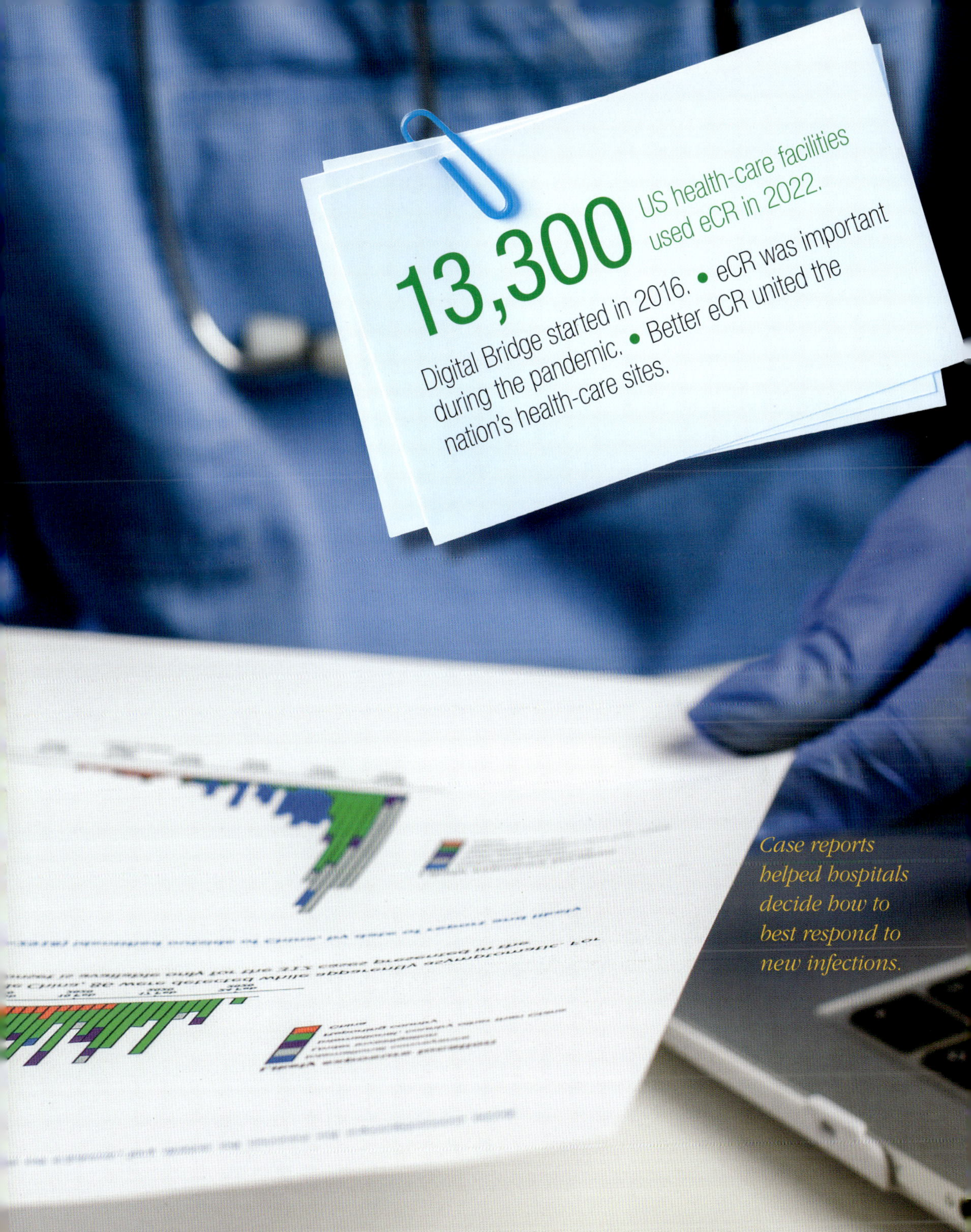

13,300 US health-care facilities used eCR in 2022.

Digital Bridge started in 2016. • eCR was important during the pandemic. • Better eCR united the nation's health-care sites.

Case reports helped hospitals decide how to best respond to new infections.

reported real-time infection. So health-care workers could manage the illness better. eCR also guided response efforts. For example, it helped decide isolation practices.

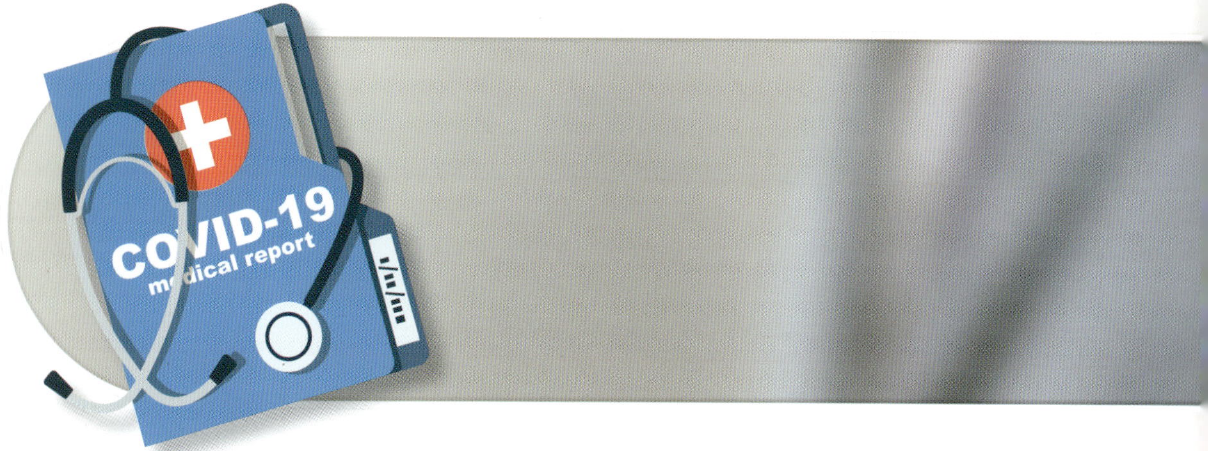

Not all health-care sites had eCR. Some health-care sites reported cases by hand. This was a problem. It was slow. Some reports were never written or collected. Cerner is a technology company in Missouri. It works with health-care information. Cerner saw a need for better eCR. In early 2021, it made a national eCR system. This helped link health-care sites. Now health-care workers could focus on the patient instead of paperwork. The new system united the nation. All health-care teams could see the reports. They had better control over COVID-19.

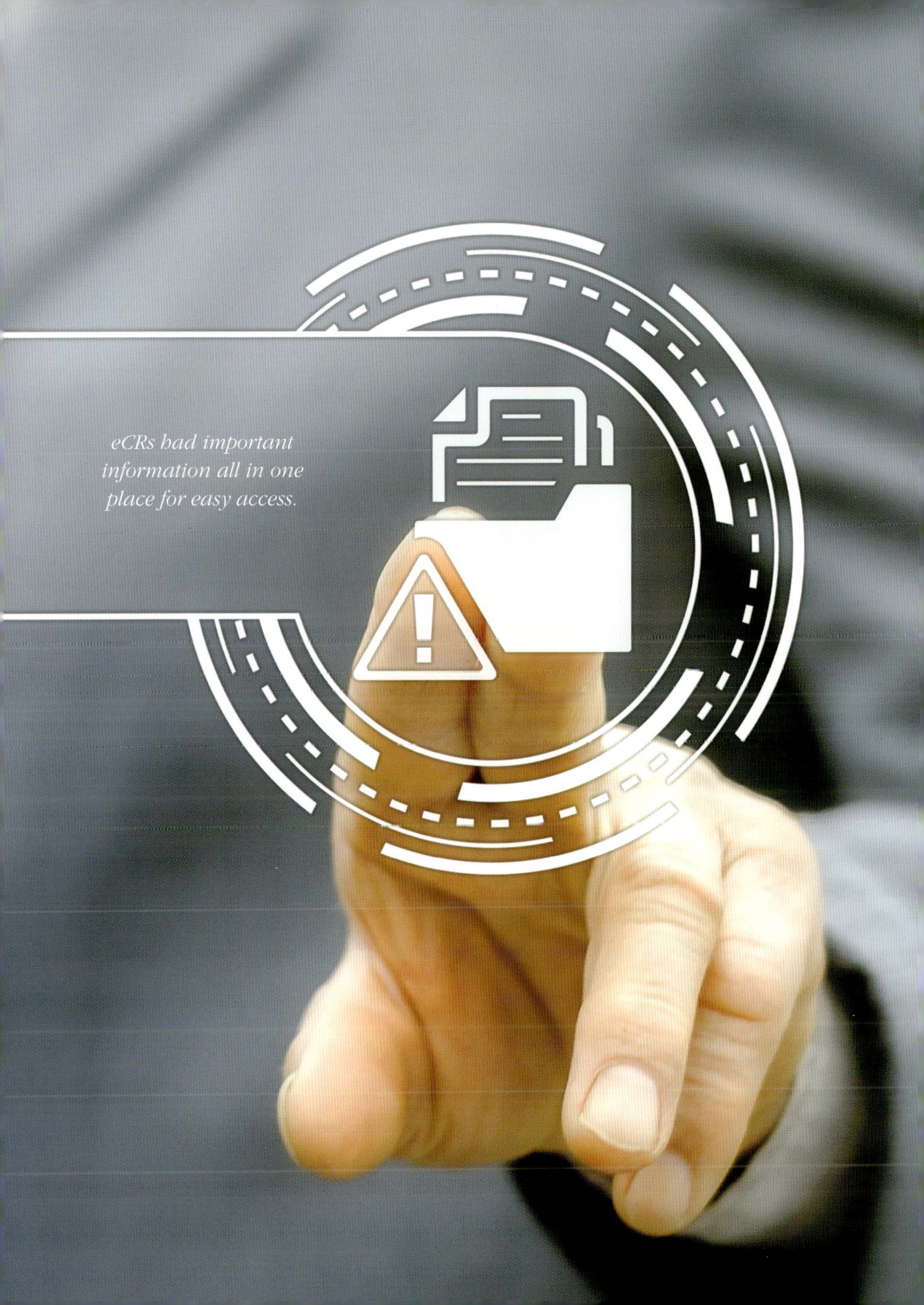
eCRs had important information all in one place for easy access.

Apps Help Manage *Spread*

10

Contact tracing is an important process. It tells who has been infected. It finds and notifies who has been in contact with them. In this way, it traces the spread of the illness. Contact tracing helps people protect themselves and others. It does not stop the spread altogether. But it helps to slow it.

Before COVID-19, contact tracing was mostly done by hand. Health-care workers led interviews. They took information about a person's illness. They discussed who came in contact with them. COVID-19 changed contact tracing. Interviews were no longer done by hand. Instead, a smartphone was used.

Singapore started using this technology for COVID-19. TraceTogether was launched in March 2020. It was the first main COVID-19 tracking app. It can tell what phones have been close together. It helped in contact tracing. In Singapore, all COVID-19 cases are reported to the Ministry

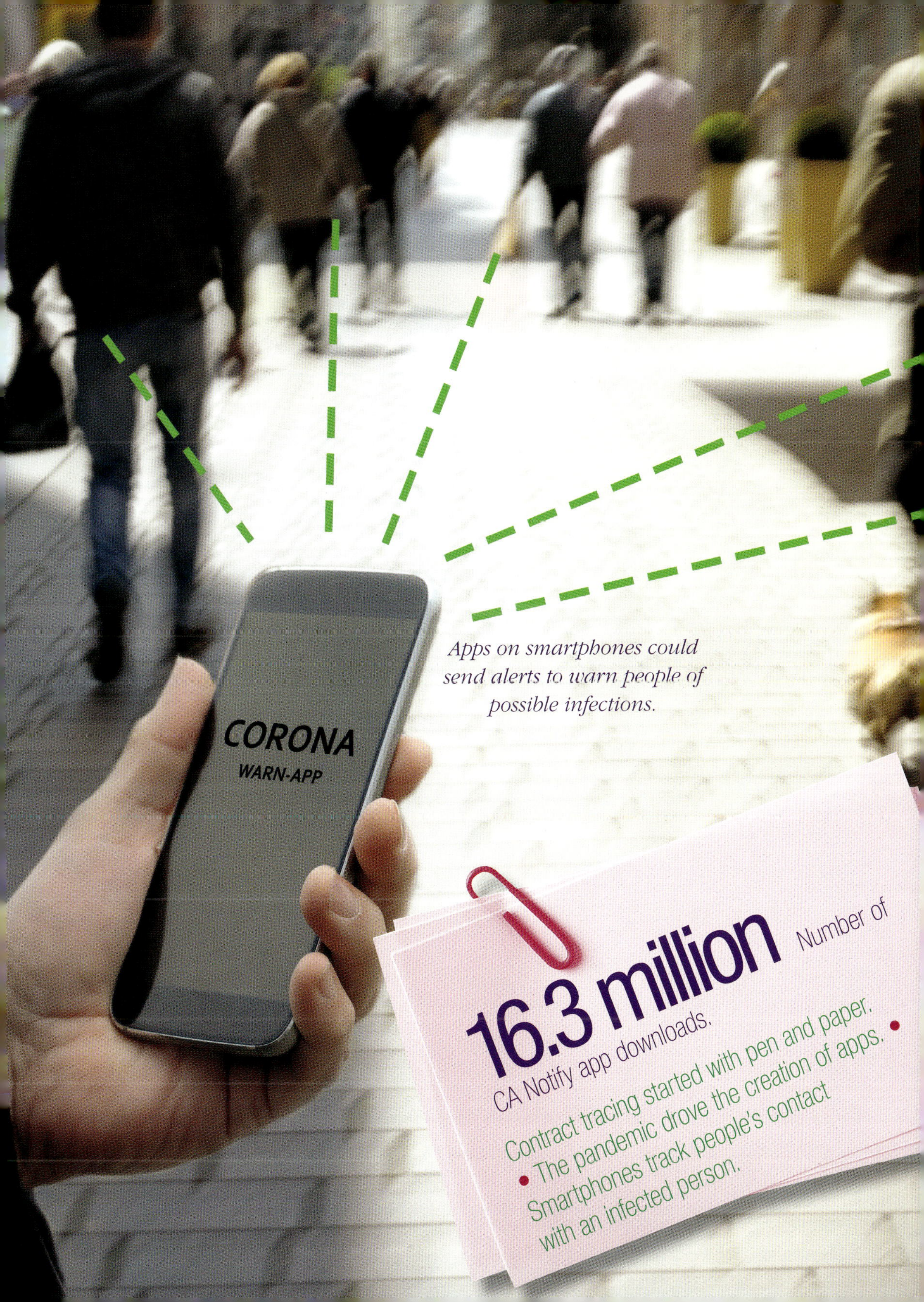

Apps on smartphones could send alerts to warn people of possible infections.

16.3 million Number of CA Notify app downloads.

Contract tracing started with pen and paper. • The pandemic drove the creation of apps. • Smartphones track people's contact with an infected person.

of Health. It is a government organization. It is in charge of the health-care system. When a case came in, the organization used the app. They sent a message to all users who were in close contact with the infected person. Then those people could choose to self-isolate. A quick response helped Singapore keep infection rates low.

Around the same time, Apple and Google went to work. They develop electronics and software. Together, they made application programming interfaces (APIs). An API allows two applications to talk to each other. The goal was to help with contact tracing. It mainly connected Android and iOS devices. Their main API was the Exposure Notifications System. This system alerts a user if they have been in contact with someone with COVID-19. Like TraceTogether, it uses Bluetooth signals. The Bluetooth does not record someone's exact location. Instead, it records people who have been near each other.

Dr. Christopher Longhurst also worked on an app. He increased the use of app contact tracing in California. His app is called CA Notify. It was released in December 2020.

Think About It In 2022, a study was done. It looked at worldwide contact tracing efforts. It found that most countries did little to no COVID-19 contact tracing. Why do you think this is?

Medications Treat and Prevent *COVID-19*

11

Gilead is a California company. It does medical research. Gilead made a medicine in 2009. It is called Veklury. It was used to fight viruses like the COVID-19. Researchers started a trial in 2020. They tested Veklury with 2,043 COVID-19 patients. The patients were from 17 countries. The medicine was injected into the patient. It stopped genetic material from replicating. Veklury worked best for patients who got it soon after infection. It lowered the risk of going to the hospital by 87 percent. By the end of 2020, the FDA approved it for general use. It was the first COVID-19 medicine.

Pfizer is a medical company in New York. It has worked on medications since 1849. It made a medicine for COVID-19 called Paxlovid. A **clinical trial** was done. More than 2,000 patients took three pills. The pills stopped a protein of the virus. The virus could

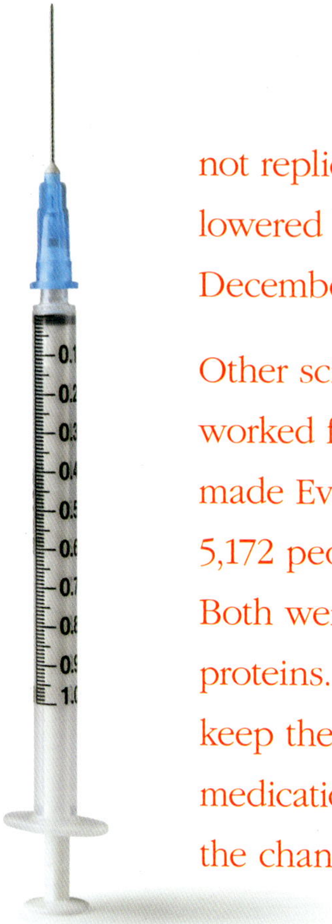

not replicate. The risk of becoming severely ill was lowered by 89 percent. The FDA approved Paxlovid in December 2021.

Other scientists wanted a medicine for prevention. They worked for AstraZeneca in the United Kingdom. They made Evusheld in December 2021. Its clinical trial had 5,172 people. The medicine was given in two doses. Both were injections. The medicine is made of lab-made proteins. The proteins boost the immune system. They keep the virus from connecting to human cells. The medication helped most people in the trial. It lowered the chance of getting COVID-19.

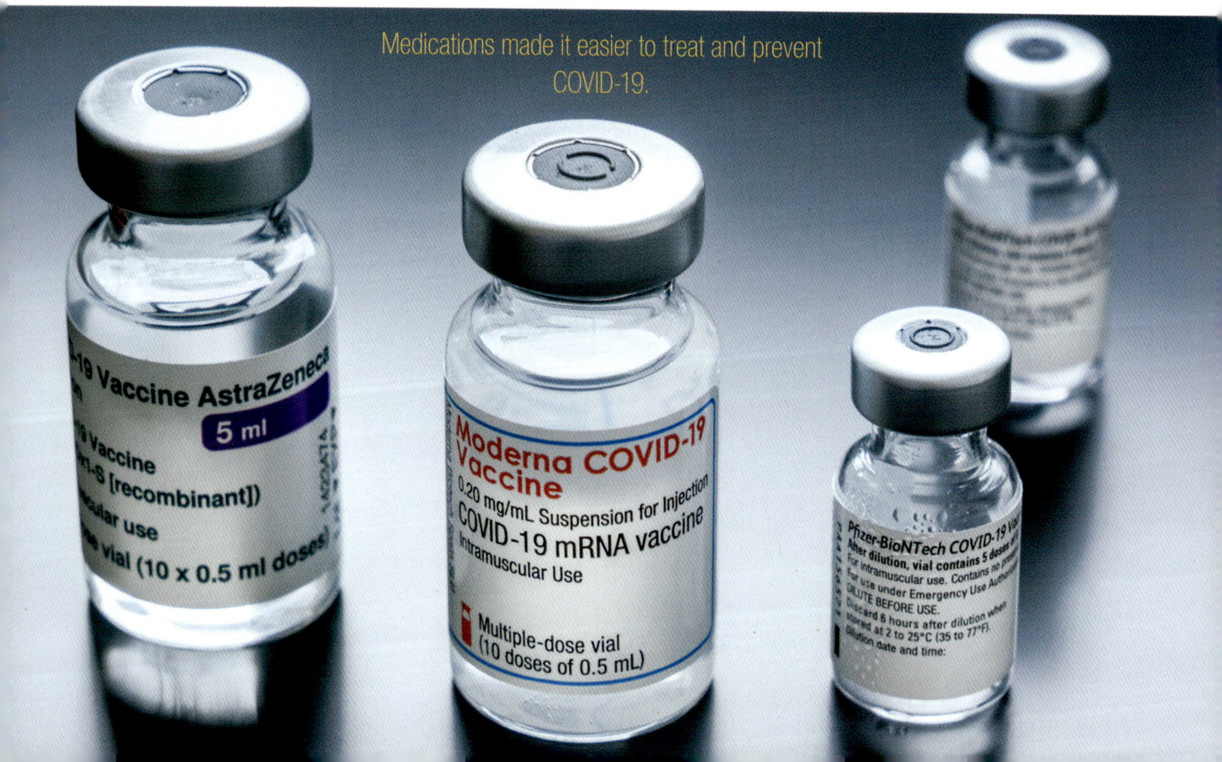

Medications made it easier to treat and prevent COVID-19.

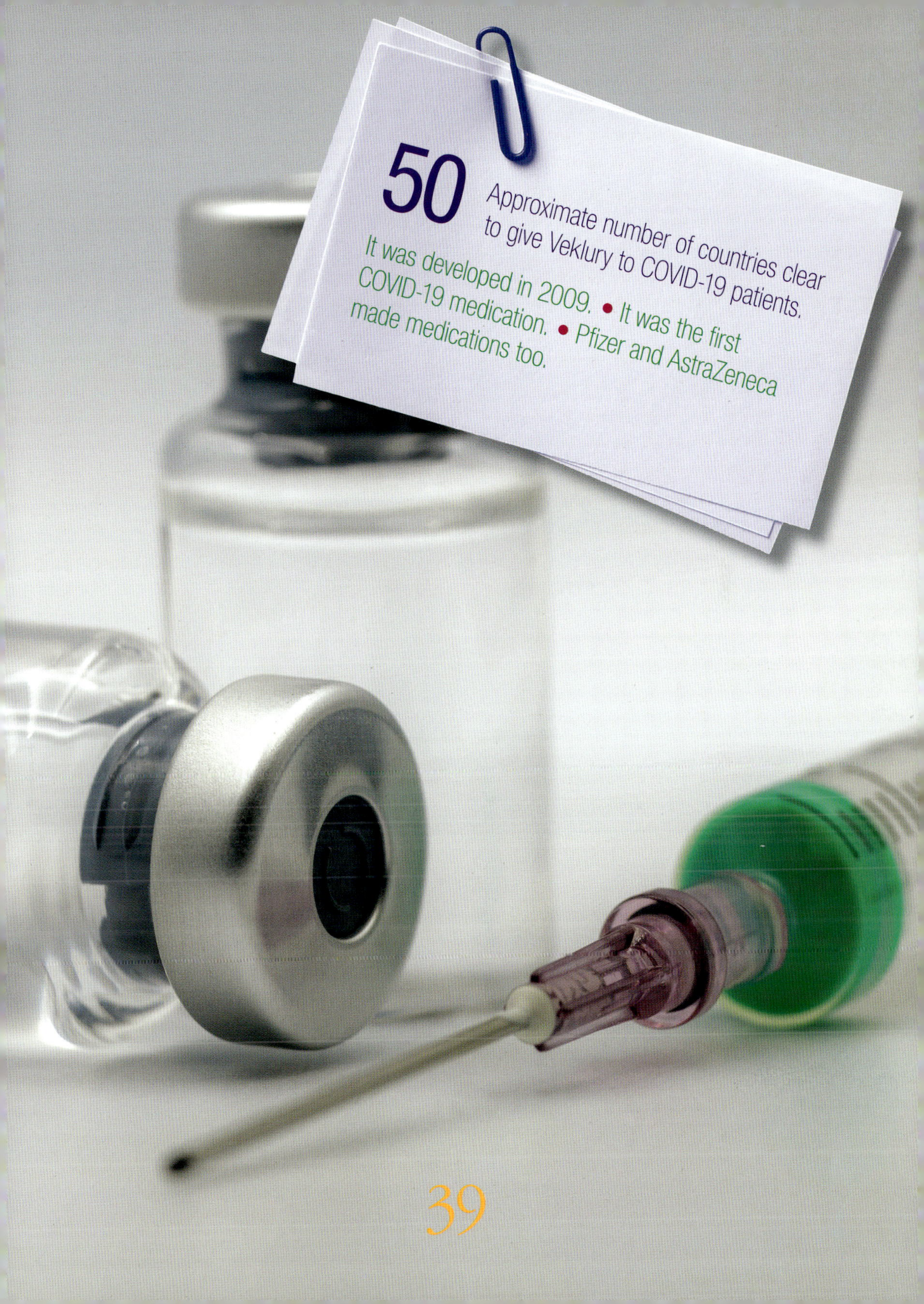

50 Approximate number of countries clear to give Veklury to COVID-19 patients.

It was developed in 2009. • It was the first COVID-19 medication. • Pfizer and AstraZeneca made medications too.

mRNA Vaccines Developed in *Record Time*

12

mRNA is an important molecule. It carries messages from the cell's DNA. The "m" stands for messenger. Scientists studied mRNA for many years. It was used to make a **vaccine** for Ebola.

Ebola is caused by a virus. Scientists thought mRNA could be used for the COVID-19 too. They made a vaccine quickly. The COVID-19 vaccine has mRNA. The mRNA enters the person's body. It tells cells how to make a protein. The protein works with the immune system. Antibodies are made. They defend against COVID-19. Two companies made the first vaccine. One is Pfizer. The other is BioNTech.

The vaccine was tested on people. The trial lasted from July 2020 to January 2021. There were three phases. The first two phases tested people of different ages.

mRNA CHALLENGES

mRNA vaccines were first tested on mice. This was in the 1990s. It was first tested on humans in 2013. Between those years, scientists faced a challenge. The mRNA did not last in the body. It couldn't deliver its message. So scientists worked on protecting the mRNA. They found that fatty droplets protected it. Now the mRNA could deliver its message.

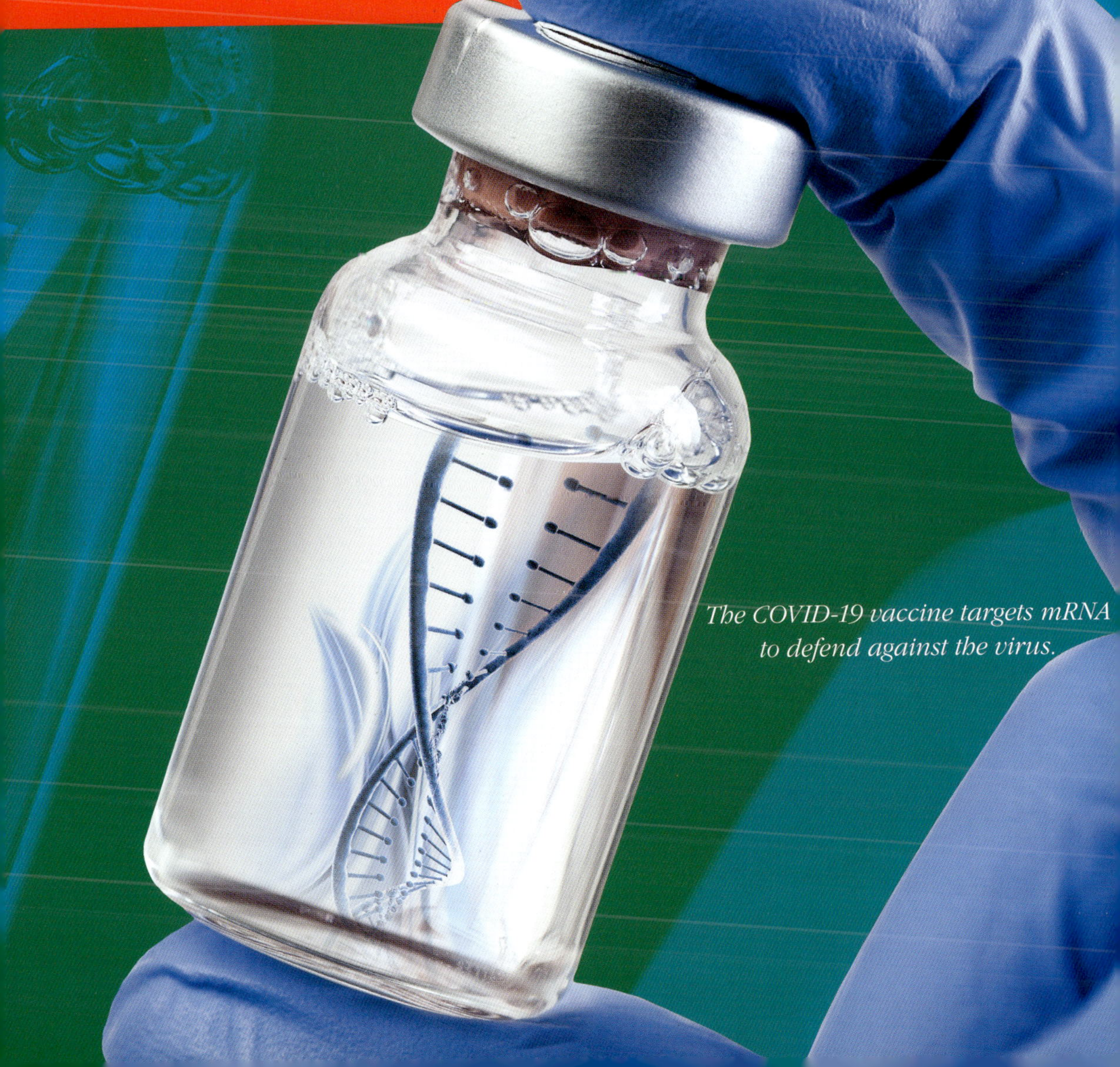

The COVID-19 vaccine targets mRNA to defend against the virus.

Phase three tested the vaccine against a **placebo**. There were 46,331 people in the trial. The FDA approved the vaccine. Another mRNA vaccine was made. The company Moderna made it. It was approved in 2022.

Johnson & Johnson also makes vaccines. It made a different one for COVID-19. This one does not use mRNA. It is a viral-vector vaccine. This technology has existed since the 1970s. It is used for most vaccines. The vaccine uses a vector virus. It is not the virus that causes COVID-19. The vector virus tells cells to make a protein. The protein teaches cells how to respond to the virus. The body makes antibodies. This builds a person's immune system. Then the body can fight COVID-19. This vaccine was tested on 39,321 people. Two of three trial phases were done. The FDA cleared the vaccine for emergency use in 2021.

6 Months to complete the three-phase vaccine trial.

mRNA carries DNA messages. • It was used to quickly create a COVID-19 vaccine. • The FDA approved multiple vaccines.

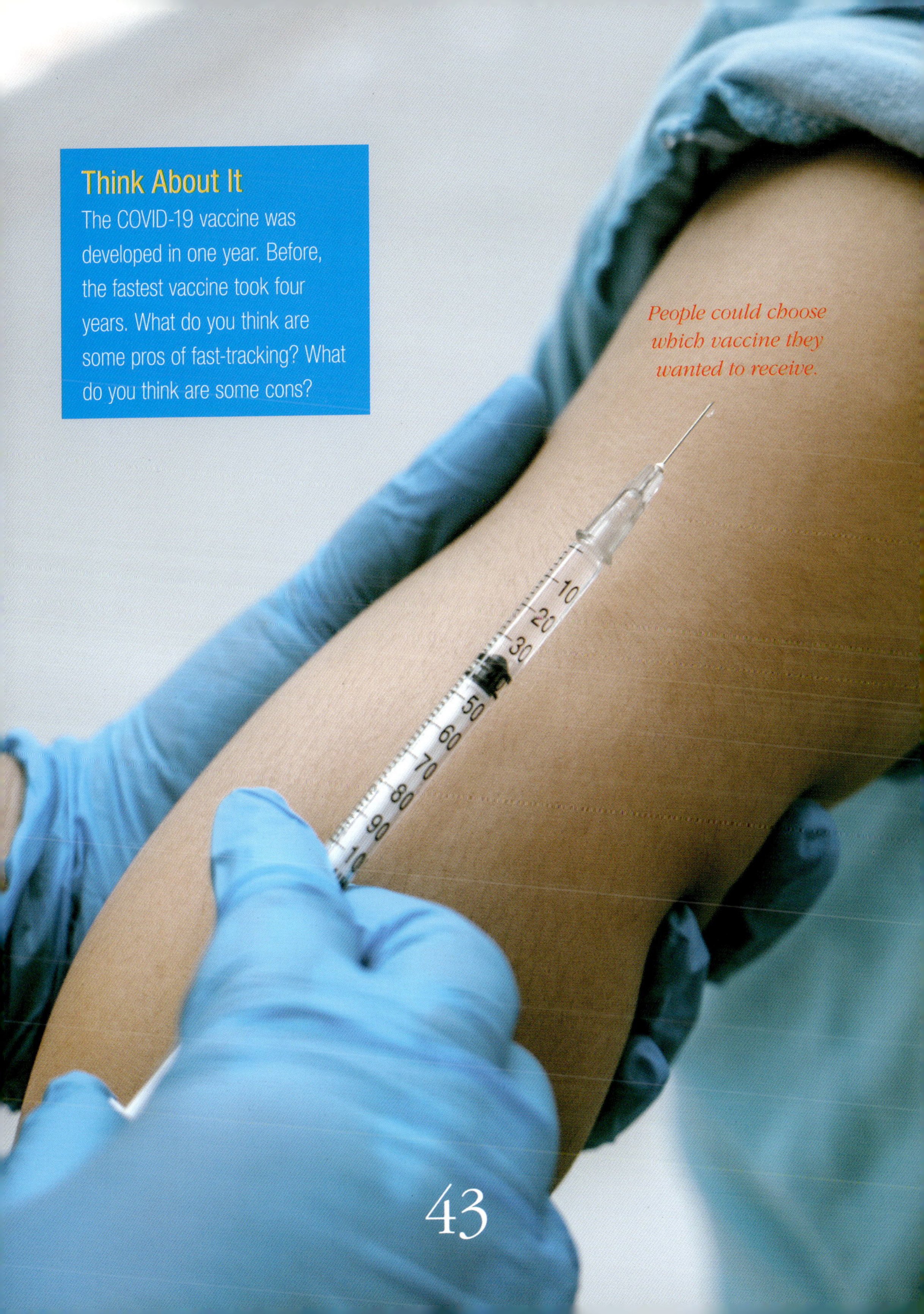

Think About It

The COVID-19 vaccine was developed in one year. Before, the fastest vaccine took four years. What do you think are some pros of fast-tracking? What do you think are some cons?

People could choose which vaccine they wanted to receive.

Fact Sheet

• Dr. Kary B. Mullis won the Nobel Prize in 1993. It was for the PCR approach. It changed science forever. Before, it took weeks to study DNA. With the PCR approach, it takes hours. It is even used to study crime scenes. It helps identify DNA evidence. This can show who did the crime.

• COVID-19 antibody tests fall into three categories. The first test is a qualitative test. This test reports if antibodies are present. The second test is a semi-quantitative test. This test reports antibody levels. The third test is a quantitative test. This test also reports antibody levels. Antibody levels can help explain how a person's body will fight COVID-19.

• Clinical trials are done to test a vaccine. Pfizer tested the first COVID-19 vaccine. The trial helped decide the dose for different age groups. The company used 153 worldwide trial sites. The trial began in July 2020. The vaccine was approved 13 months later.

• Face masks appeared at Paris' Fashion Week in February 2020. It was the beginning of the COVID-19 outbreak. Fashion designer Marine Serre was the creator. She designed masks that went with her outfits.

• Early on in the COVID-19 pandemic, current infections were tracked. Public health groups counted completed tests. Results were also reported.

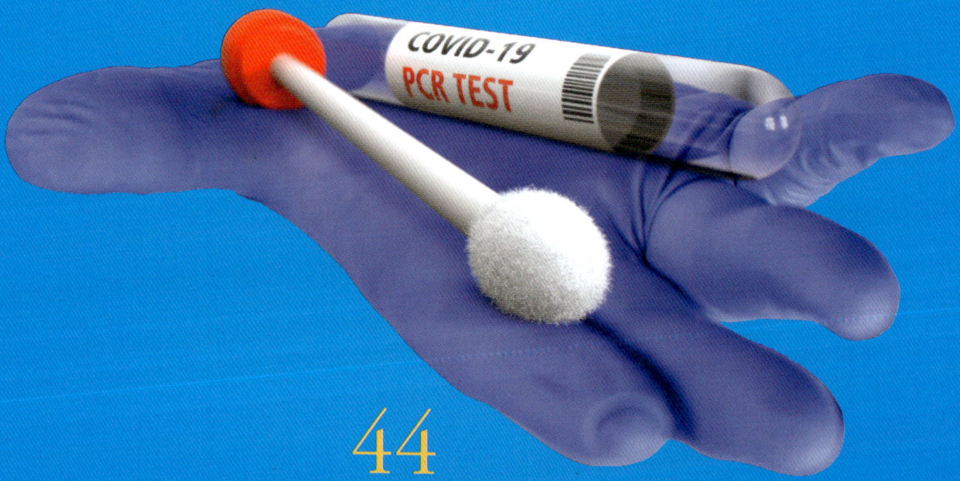

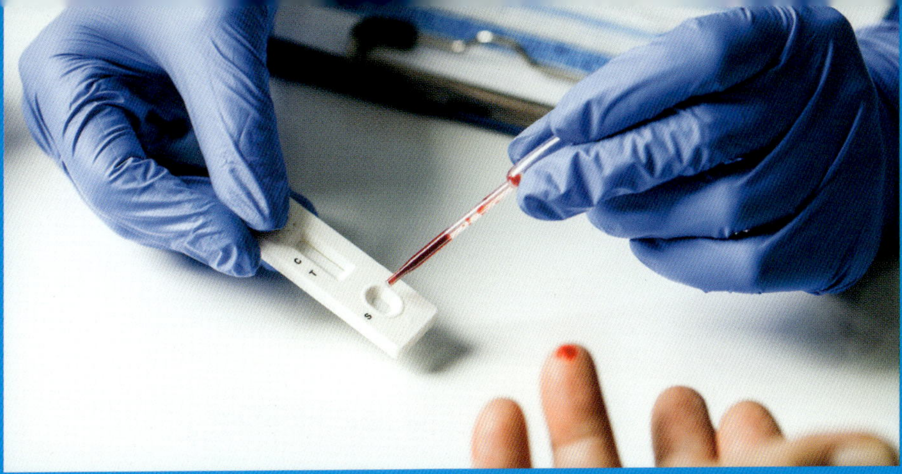

By August 2020, a total of 79,611,982 tests had been done in the the United States. Of those tests, about 9 percent recorded positive results.

- Dr. Forrest Bird had an early interest in aviation. It led him to his first solo flight in 1935. He was 14 years old. Later, he entered the Army Air Corp. He flew all kinds of aircraft. During a flight, he used a breathing device. He grew curious about it. It led him to medical school. Then Bird founded Percussionaire in 1983. It focused on making ventilation devices.

- COVID-19 vaccines and booster shots are widely available. But vaccine breakthrough infections have happened. This means a fully vaccinated person still gets sick with COVID-19. No COVID-19 vaccine prevents illness 100 percent of the time. From January to November 2021, breakthroughs were studied. About 1 in 100 fully vaccinated people still got COVID-19. It was most common for people with weakened immune systems.

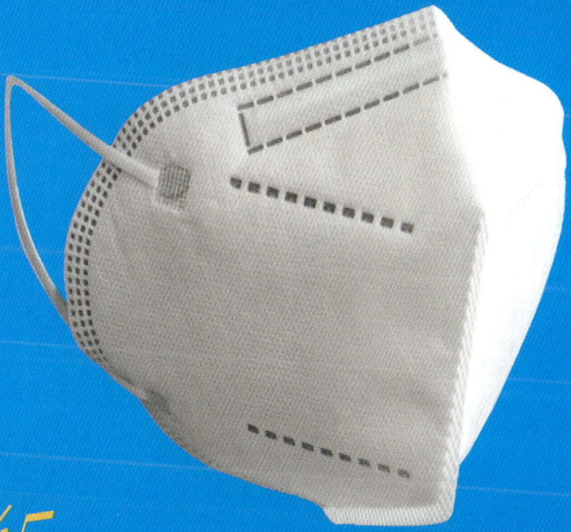

Glossary

antibody
A substance made by the body to fight disease or toxic materials.

antigen
A substance that causes the body to have an immune reaction and make antibodies.

bellows
A tool that sends a gust of air out when its sides are pushed in.

clinical trial
A research study of volunteers and the safety/effectiveness of a vaccine.

diagnose
To pinpoint a disease or illness in someone.

fiberglass
A material made up of tiny threads of glass.

genetic
Having to do with the material in the body that is in charge of a person's physical traits and characteristics that get passed from one generation to the next.

immunity
The power to resist a disease or illness.

mass-produced
Made in a large quantity, usually by a machine.

pandemic
A disease or illness that spreads fast and affects a large number of people in the world.

placebo
A substance that does not affect disease; used as a control in testing new drugs.

plasma
A substance that is similar to a gas but that can carry electricity.

polio
A serious disease that damages nerves of the spine and can lead to someone becoming paralyzed.

polymer
A chemical compound made up of small molecules that repeat in pattern, forming a larger molecule.

respirator
A device that is worn over the nose and mouth to keep someone from breathing in a harmful substance.

sterilize
To clean something by destroying germs and bacteria.

vaccine
A substance injected into a person that helps protect against a disease.

vital signs
Measurements such as heart rate, blood pressure, and temperature that can be tracked to help determine a person's health.

For More Information

Books

Cross, Paul Ian. *How to Vanquish a Virus.* London: Welbeck Publishing Group, 2022.

Hanel, Rachael. *The COVID Pandemic.* Mankato, MN: Creative Education/Creative Paperbacks, 2023.

Sommer, Nathan. *The Coronavirus Pandemic.* Minneapolis: Bellwether Media, 2022.

Websites

Beat the Germs! Game
https://vaxpackhero.com/

Coronavirus Glossary
https://kids.nationalgeographic.com/science/article/coronavirus-glossary

 • Top Rank is an imprint of Black Rabbit Books. • Edited by Book Buddy Media | Designed by Danny Nanos • Photographs © Alamy: Sabena Jane Blackbird, 12; Dreamstime Motortion, 8–9, Mykola Pokhodzhay, 16, Paul Vinten, 20; Shutterstock: Andrey_Popov, 10, 45, Andy Dean Photography, 8, Anterovium, 38, Belinda Pretorius, 48, beton studio, 7, Billion Photos cover, 2–3, Chot Studio, 43, Cryptographer, 26, 45, 30–31, 40–41, Giovanni Cancemi, 4, 44, HenadziPechan, 26, hvostik, 32–33, Immersion Imagery, 34, Ink Drop, 27, 28–29, Jarun Ontakrai, 25, Jolygon, 46–47, Joshua Jay Koppelman, 14–15, KPG-Ivary, 4–5, Limbitech, 6, Lunx, 13, Marc Bruxelle, 38, Maren Winter, 35, Michael Vi, 27, Mongta Studio, 36, My Ocean Production, 19, Nao Novoa, 5, Panchenko Vladimir, 32–33, Pavel L Photo and Video, 11, Prostock-studio, 22, 23, RAJ CREATIONZS, 17, SB Arts Media, 17, 20, Scott Maxwell LuMaxArt, 21, Tridsanu Thopet, 21, Wut_Moppie, 37, 39 • Printed in China

Library of Congress Cataloging-in-Publication Data is filed under LCCN 2023052891. ISBN 9781645823001 (library binding), ISBN 9781645823322 (paperback), ISBN 9781645823643 (ebook)

Index

About the Author

Janie Scheffer is a former classroom teacher and current educational writer. She has taught first grade, a postgraduate reading methods course, and many grade levels in between. She specializes in literacy instruction and writing for the K–8 audience. She has written literacy curricula, literacy assessments, educational articles, blog posts, and, most recently, children's books.